The Prostate Answer Book:

Remedies and Cures for Every Man and What Your Doctor Never Tells You About Surgery

Publisher's Note

This book is for information only and is not intended to be a medical guide for self-diagnosis or self-treatment. It does not constitute medical advice and should not be construed as such or used in place of your doctor's medical advice. We recommend in all cases that you contact your personal doctor or health care provider before taking or discontinuing any medication, or before treating yourself in any way.

While every attempt has been made to assure that the information in this book is true and accurate, errors may occur; and it is not possible to cover every symptom, condition, and treatment. The publisher, editors, and medical advisor disclaim all liability in connection with the use of the information in this book.

"Blessed is the man who finds wisdom, the man who gains understanding, for she is more profitable than silver, and yields better returns than gold."

— Proverbs 3:13-14

First printing April 2003

ISBN 1-890957-03-8

Contents

About our medical advisor

J. Curtis Nickel, M.D., F.R.C.S.C., D.A.B.U.
Professor, Department of Urology
Queen's University
Staff Urologist, Department of Urology
Kingston General and Hotel Dieu Hospitals
Kingston, Ontario, Canada

Dr. Nickel was born, educated, and completed his undergraduate, surgical, urological, and research training in Canada. He has been a member of the Department of Urology at Queen's University since 1984 and was promoted to full professor in 1994.

Dr. Nickel's research has been in the fields of inflammatory diseases of the urinary tract and diseases of the prostate gland. He has written over 150 scientific papers, reviews, chapters, and books on these subjects. He maintains a laboratory at Queen's University, funded continuously by peer reviewed and industry grants, including grants from the U.S. National Institutes of Health. Dr. Nickel's clinical research prostate center is supported in part with a R-01 (DK53746-01) grant from the U.S. National Institutes of Health/National Institute of Diabetes and Digestive and Kidney Diseases.

He participates as organizer, chairman, invited lecturer, or visiting professor in many local, national, and international university and CME events. He has given lectures in over 25 countries. He is on the scientific or review panel of numerous granting agencies, a regular reviewer for many urological and medical journals, a member of the Canadian Prostate Health Council, and is the only foreign member of the American Board of Urology Examination Committee.

List of illustrations

Just the facts, Ma'am.
Joe Friday, *Dragnet*

Introduction:
A closer look at the facts

Think prostate problems spell certain death for any sort of sex life? Well, think again. Some prostate problems are actually caused by too little sex.

That's just one of the many misconceptions men have about the prostate. In fact, of all the organs in a man's body, the prostate is the most misunderstood. Younger men commonly think only older men have prostate problems. Other men aren't even aware of that mysterious gland until it starts giving them problems.

Unfortunately, many of these misunderstandings about the prostate come disguised in the form of facts. It's all too easy to generalize and sensationalize a simple fact into something else entirely. As you'll see in the following examples, that's why it always pays to take a closer look at so-called facts, especially really scary ones. Sometimes, the difference between life and death or health and happiness is just a mismanaged, misquoted, misunderstood fact.

Fact: This year the American Cancer Society estimates that 209,900 men will be diagnosed with prostate cancer and 41,800 men will die from prostate cancer. Those figures have risen steadily since 1973. They rose even faster in the 1980s after the prostate specific antigen (PSA) test to detect prostate cancer was introduced. In fact, figures from the National Cancer Institute suggest that the incidence of prostate cancer has risen 176 percent since 1973.

A closer look: All those numbers might lead you to believe that prostate cancer is on the rise — that your exit in life will probably be with the prostate cancer parade. A closer look at the data reveals the numbers really don't add up that way. What's really on the rise is the *detection* of prostate cancer. In fact, those numbers follow a path similar to breast cancer rates after mammograms were introduced in the mid-1970s. First rates go up, then they decrease, and finally they level off. The most recent research says the new cases of prostate cancer detected each year appear to be falling.

Fact: Prostate cancer is the most common cancer in men, after skin cancer.

A closer look: Although prostate cancer is an extremely common cancer in men, it is not the leading cancer killer of men — that distinction falls to lung cancer. In fact, prostate cancer is fairly uncommon in men under 50. Plus, most prostate cancers are slow-growing, so even if you're diagnosed with cancer, you have a good chance of dying with and not from it — in other words, you'll probably die of something other than prostate cancer.

Fact: Symptoms such as difficulty urinating, frequent urination, and dribbling are suggestive of benign prostatic hyperplasia (BPH).

A closer look: Other diseases or even taking certain kinds of decongestants can cause symptoms very similar to BPH. That's why it's important that your doctor take a careful medical history, do a thorough physical exam, and use the appropriate laboratory tests to rule out a urethral stricture (narrowing of the urethra), bladder irritation, cancer, or stones before diagnosing BPH. Experts estimate that as many as 30 percent of the men who undergo surgery for BPH show no evidence of BPH once the surgeon slices open the prostate.

Since facts aren't always as clear as they may seem, you can use this book to help you wade through the ocean of information to find the pearls of wisdom that can really make a difference to your health. When you know what the doctor is talking about, you're more prepared to ask the right questions and choose the treatment option that's best for you.

How to use this book

In this book, you'll find the most up-to-date information on a variety of prostate problems to help you make informed decisions about your health. Chapters 1 through 6 contain an overview of the prostate, as well as an in-depth look at the most common prostate problems and treatments. Charts and checklists help give you insight into your prostate difficulties so you can discuss problems more productively with your doctor. Easy-to-understand diagrams clearly explain all your treatment options and give you pointers for picking the treatment most suited for you.

The prevention of prostate cancer is the focus of Chapter 7. Some researchers estimate that up to 70 percent of all prostate cancers may be preventable. In this chapter, you'll find out how to minimize your risk of prostate cancer. Since regular screening tests are an important part of this process, they are clearly explained in Chapter 8.

Chapters 9, 10, and 11 deal with the diagnosis of cancer and common treatments. Nutrition and other natural therapies are discussed, as well as treatment options for advanced prostate cancer. You'll also find suggestions for handling the emotional and psychological aspects of cancer.

The most common side effects from treating prostate problems, both cancerous and noncancerous, are covered in Chapters 12 and 13. Coping with incontinence or impotence becomes easier once you know that a large number of treatment options can help you manage both conditions effectively.

You may notice that doctors are referred to as "he" throughout the book. This is simply for ease of reading. This doesn't intend to suggest that male doctors are preferred over female doctors. You should always choose the doctor (whether female or male) best qualified to treat your particular problems.

In each chapter, you will find that any tests used for diagnosing your condition are arranged according to the order in which each test is likely to be performed. This order usually progresses from simple tests to more complex exams. Chapter 14 offers a more detailed explanation of all the different diagnostic tests you may encounter.

Each chapter closes with a section called "In summary." It is a brief summary of all the important points covered in that chapter.

Several other chapters of the book offer additional information you may find helpful. These include an overview of different prostate medicines and possible side effects and a list of support groups and organizations you can contact for more information.

A bibliography of sources used for this book will give you some good ideas for further reading. And last, but certainly not least, is the invaluable index — the best way to find specific information fast.

* * * * *

We hope this book helps dispel the myths and clarify the facts about this complex organ in a friendly, readable way. Godspeed your quest for good health!

The Editors of FC&A

Things should be as simple as possible but not any simpler.
Albert Einstein, American physicist

1

Your healthy prostate

The word prostate was originally derived from the Greek word prohistani, meaning to stand in front of. Supposedly Herophilus of Alexandria came up with the word in 335 B.C. when he used it to describe an organ located in front of the bladder. (Actually, it's more under the bladder than in front of it, but that's not bad for 2,000 some years ago.)

For about 2,272 years, that was all anyone knew about the prostate. Only in the past 60 years have doctors begun to determine the purpose of the prostate and uncover a little about the problems that tend to pester this small but important gland.

A tour of the prostate gland

Picture a walnut. That's just about the size and shape of your prostate. Normally the size of a pea when you're born, it stays that way until puberty. Then, hormones stimulate your prostate's growth until it reaches its adult size, when you're around age 20. It stays that size until about age 25 when it starts to grow again. By about age 50, this continued growth can add up to urination difficulties. Although the full-grown prostate only weighs about an ounce, it probably gives men more problems than any other organ in the body.

The adult prostate consists of muscles, fibrous tissue, and glands. The prostate is not really one large gland but rather a grape-like cluster of small glands called acini. You have between 20 and 60 acini bunches in your prostate, each of which connects to the urethra (the tube that transports urine and semen to the

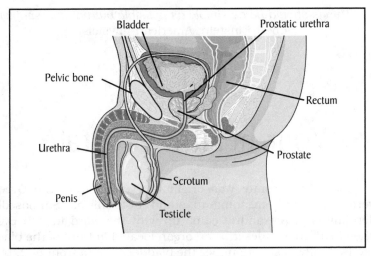

Figure 1.1 - The prostate gland and nearby structures.

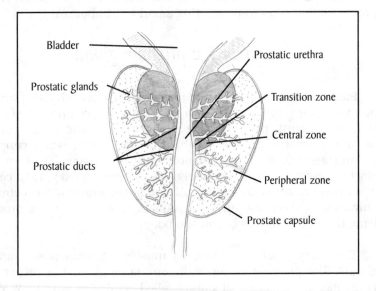

Figure 1.2 - The zones of the prostate.

penis and out of the body). The entire prostate is enclosed in muscular tissue called the prostatic capsule.

The glandular part of the prostate is divided into three zones: the peripheral zone, the transition zone, and the central zone. The peripheral zone makes up the majority of the prostate. The central zone is the second-largest part. The transition zone is the smallest area, making up only 5 to 10 percent of the entire gland. The differences between these zones is relatively hard to see unless the prostate is not healthy.

Benign prostatic hyperplasia (BPH) occurs mostly in the transition zone. Cancer usually shows up in the peripheral zone, although it can affect the other two zones as well.

The prostate puzzle

By the time you hit puberty, you probably thought you knew all you needed to know about your prostate. According to an article in the March 26, 1995, edition of the London Times, the majority of men don't know as much as they might think.

The Times survey revealed that 89 percent of men don't know where the prostate is located, and 62 percent got the prostate confused with the bladder. Only half of the men knew women didn't have prostates, too.

If you too are in a puzzle over your prostate, read on to find out just how those puzzling prostate pieces fit together.

The prostate's purpose

Unlike the appendix (which some doctors say has no apparent purpose), the prostate really does have a purpose. A part of the male reproductive system, its primary job is to produce some of the fluid that carries sperm.

The prostate is where fluid produced by the seminal vesicles and testicles mixes with fluid produced by the prostate. This fluid vehicle is what provides transportation and protection for sperm. That makes your prostate sort of like your body's own bus system — the prostate is the hub where all the buses leave from.

However, unlike a normal bus system, the prostate's buses never come back so it has to continually create new ones. Since the prostate secretes fluid used to transport sperm, it is considered a gland (all glands secrete something of some sort).

Just like average city buses, your prostate's buses must travel the highways and byways of your body's reproductive system to reach their final destination (your penis). The prostate gland empties its secretions into prostate ducts, which empty into the urethra. In the urethra, the secretions join up with sperm to form semen.

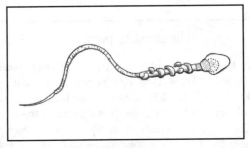

Figure 1.3 - A mature sperm. The smallest cells in your body are the sperm cells. Each measures about 1/500 of an inch. It takes about 74 days for a sperm cell to mature.

However, the prostate does not limit its influence to just the reproductive process. It also influences the male urinary system. In fact, any man who has ever suffered with BPH would probably say the prostate puts quite a squeeze on the urinary system.

That's due to the prostate's strategic location. (Some men say it's conveniently situated to give a man as many problems as possible.) The prostate sits due south of the bladder. It surrounds the top part of the urethra. If the prostate enlarges or gets irritated, the urethra is often the organ that suffers the most.

To understand how the prostate affects both the reproductive and urinary systems, the following quick guides and illustrations will give you a clear idea of what part the prostate plays in each.

User's guide to the reproductive system

For a quick review of the male reproductive system, start at the bottom (with the scrotum) and work your way up, around, and back down. That's basically the way the system works. The accompanying illustration provides a look at each individual part and at the overall system.

Scrotum – The sac of skin that contains the testicles.

Testicles – The manufacturing plant for sperm and testosterone.

Sperm – A reproductive cell capable of fertilizing a woman's egg, which, if timing is right and conditions are good, may eventually develop into a baby. See page 8.

Epididymis – Stores mature sperm and provides nutrition to immature sperm.

Ductus (vas) deferens – The tube that carries sperm up to the prostatic urethra through muscle contractions.

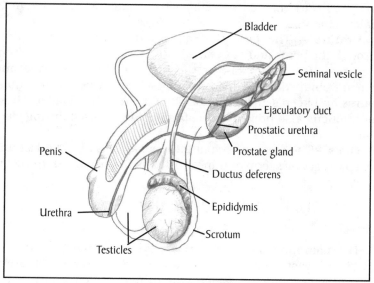

Figure I.4 - The male reproductive system.

> ### Did you know?
>
> The testicles produce 10 million new sperm cells every day. In only 18 months, one man can produce enough sperm cells (over 5 billion) to populate the entire world. A single ejaculation can produce up to 500 million sperm, all contained in barely a teaspoonful of semen.

Seminal vesicles – Small sacs connected to the ductus deferens that produce nutrient-rich secretions that combine with sperm to make semen.

Ejaculatory ducts – The channel formed by the ductus deferens and the seminal vesicle, which joins the prostatic urethra.

Prostatic urethra – The part of the urethra completely encircled by the prostate gland.

Prostate gland – The part-muscle, part-gland structure that produces nutrient-rich secretions that combine with sperm to make semen.

Urethra – The tube that carries urine from the bladder through the penis and out of the body. It also carries semen from the prostatic urethra out of the body. To prevent urine and semen from mixing, bladder neck muscles contract during intercourse and keep semen from backing up into the bladder. These contractions also prevent urine from being released during ejaculation.

Penis – The organ of sexual intercourse. It is also the last and final passageway sperm or urine must pass through to exit the body.

User's guide to the urinary system

The main function of your urinary system is to help your body get rid of waste products by creating and disposing of urine. Unlike the reproductive system, the urinary system starts at the top (with the kidneys) and works its way down. The accompanying illustration, found on page 13, provides a look at each individual part and at the overall system.

Kidneys – This is where urine formation begins. Urine is formed as your body breaks down the food you eat into chemical byproducts. These leftovers are transported by your bloodstream to the kidneys. The kidneys then filter your blood to collect the waste and excess water, forming urine.

Ureters – These tubes, attached to the center of each kidney, transport urine to the bladder.

Bladder – A muscular pouch that temporarily stores urine until it can be excreted from your body.

Volume monitors – Specialized nerves in the trigone (base of bladder) and bladder wall that monitor the amount of urine in the bladder. Once enough liquid has collected, they signal the brain that the bladder needs to be emptied.

Urethra – The tube that carries urine from the bladder through the penis and out of the body. It also carries semen from the prostatic urethra out of the body. To prevent urine and semen from becoming mixed, bladder neck muscles contract during intercourse and keep semen from backing up into the bladder. These contractions also prevent urine from being released during ejaculation.

Prostate gland – Produces nutrient-rich secretions that combine with sperm to make semen. This gland really has nothing to do with your urinary system. It's simply situated in such a strategic place that if it becomes enlarged (as it often does as men grow older), it makes urinating more and more difficult.

Prostatic urethra – The part of the urethra completely encircled by the prostate gland.

Did you know?

Each of your kidneys has about 1 million separate filters. Both kidneys, working together, filter about 2.2 pints of blood per minute.

External urethral sphincter – The muscle that men use to control the release of urine.

Penis – The organ of sexual intercourse. It is also the last and final passageway sperm or urine must pass through to exit the body.

Testosterone triggers

Testosterone levels peak around sunrise. That accounts for the frequent morning erections most men have experienced.

Other activities that raise testosterone levels:

- Fighting
- TV violence
- Thinking about or actually having sex
- Winning a sports event
- A successful outcome of some sort
- Intense emotions

The mechanics of an erection

There be three things which are too wonderful for me,
yea four which I know not:
The way of an eagle in the air; the way of a serpent upon a
rock; the way of a ship in the midst of the sea;
and the way of a man with a maid.
Proverbs 30:18-19

Even today, doctors still haven't completely unraveled the mystery of the way of a man with a maid. However, they do know that an erection depends on a delicate balance of several systems within your body, including the blood vessels, nervous system, and hormones. Your mind also plays an important part.

Your blood vessels and nervous system need to be in good condition to move the amount of blood from your body into your penis

Did prostate problems provoke World War II?

Can prostate health affect the fate of nations?

Although it may seem far-fetched, some historians think prostate problems could have caused World War II.

They argue that because of poor prostate health (causing a frequent need to urinate), the heads of state did not sit still long enough to make sound treaty decisions, thus laying the groundwork for the second world war.

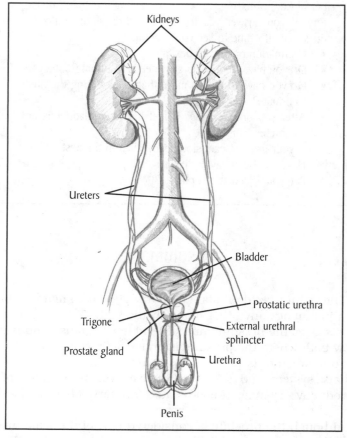

Figure 1.5 — The male urinary system.

that is required to maintain an erection — it's about 11 times the amount of blood normally found in the penis. Hormones help decide whether you have any interest in sex or not. They also influence the penis's ability to become erect. Your mind is the final factor. A mind preoccupied with anxious or stressful thoughts makes it practically impossible for the penis to perform.

Signs your prostate may be sick

A sick prostate will not suffer in silence. It has any number of ways of letting you know it's feeling less than satisfactory. If you answer yes to one or more of the following questions, it's time to see your doctor.

- Is urination painful or hesitant?
- Do you have frequent urgent needs to urinate?
- Do you have to get up more than once during the night to urinate?
- After you urinate, does it feel like your bladder is not completely empty?
- Is your urine stream slower now than in the past?
- Have you been having less sex lately?
- Are your ejaculations painful?

In summary

The walnut-sized prostate probably gives men more problems than just about any other organ in the body. To understand all the diseases the prostate must defend itself against, you need to know both where the prostate is and exactly what it does.

Your prostate is part of two major systems of the body, the urinary system and the reproductive system. As part of the reproductive system, the prostate's primary job is to produce some of the fluid that carries sperm.

Although the prostate is considered part of the male urinary system, it doesn't help in the process of collecting or eliminating waste from the body. The prostate presents more of a problem for the urinary system than anything else. It encircles part of the urethra. This strategic location means that if the prostate becomes enlarged (as it often does as men grow older), it makes urinating more and more difficult.

In addition to becoming enlarged, the prostate is also a popular spot for infections, because once they get a grip, it's very hard to shake them loose. The prostate is also the second most common site of cancer in men, after skin cancer.

Although it may seem that this small gland has more than its fair share of problems, the good news is that all of these conditions are treatable and many are curable.

Never go to a doctor whose office plants have died.
Erma Bombeck, American humorist

2

Dealing with doctors and handling insurance issues

In 1624, English poet John Donne noted, "I observe the physician with the same diligence as he the disease."

John Donne's stance was certainly a safe practice in the 17th century when doctors were at least as likely to kill you as cure you. Even today, when medical knowledge and treatments have improved by incredible leaps and bounds, it's still sound advice. For example, a study by Harvard researchers revealed that during a one-year period, 51 percent of deaths in New York hospitals were caused by neglect.

Whether your family doctor or a urologist (a doctor who specializes in treating disorders of the urinary system and male reproductive system) handles your prostate problems, you can only protect your health and your prostate by staying actively involved in your care. That means educating yourself and asking questions.

When to see a doctor

If you've been having painful ejaculation or urination or you've noticed a need to urinate much more frequently than in the past, you probably already made an appointment with your doctor. If you haven't, you should.

What to expect on your first visit

Typically, men with prostate problems first see their family doctors. Since you'll be asked to describe exactly what's bothering you, it helps to come prepared. Following is a list of information your doctor may find useful in making a diagnosis:

▶ A two- to three-day urination diary. It will actually be very helpful for your doctor if you will note exactly when you urinated, what you had to drink beforehand, an estimate of how much you urinated, whether you had any urine leakage or accidents, what you were doing when the leakage or accident occurred, or whether the urge to urinate was extremely pressing.

▶ A list of symptoms. Note whether you've experienced any of the following: painful, urgent, or frequent urination; bladder or urethral pain; bladder pain relieved by urination; blood in your semen or urine; chills; fever; low-back pain; painful intercourse or ejaculation; pain in the perineum (the area between the penis and anus) or anal area; tiredness; reduced urine stream; problems beginning urination; difficulty emptying the bladder; waking to urinate at night; urinating only small amounts; wetting yourself.

▶ Your medical history. If you're seeing the same family doctor you've been seeing for years, this won't be necessary. However, if you've changed doctors a lot or are seeing a specialist, this information can be very helpful. You don't necessarily have to get medical records from every doctor you've ever seen. Simply list any diseases you've had diagnosed, any current medical conditions you have, medicines you're taking or have taken recently (include over-the-counter medicine), any time spent in the hospital or surgeries you've had, and any medicine or food allergies. It's especially important to tell your doctor about any food or medicine allergies you have.

▶ A summary of your recent sexual activity. Include whether you've had multiple partners, types of sexual intercourse, and types (if any) of birth control used. Also, note whether any of your typical sexual patterns have changed recently.

It's easy to get rattled and rushed in the doctor's office and almost forget the reason you're there. That's why you should write down any questions you want to ask. Don't be embarrassed about taking notes while the doctor is talking. Some men prefer to use a tape recorder, while others just take along another person as a second pair of ears.

After you've talked for a few minutes, your doctor will probably want to perform a general physical exam. If your doctor suspects that your prostate is at the root of your woes, he'll probably also want to do a rectal exam and possibly test your prostate specific antigen (PSA) levels. For more information on these tests, see Chapter 8.

Make sure you have the insurance you need

Wait! Before you make that appointment to have your doctor diagnose what you suspect could be a potential prostate problem, check your insurance.

First, do you have any? If your doctor diagnoses a condition that requires a hospital stay or surgery, you need to have insurance to protect yourself financially. You don't want to wait until after your diagnosis to try to get coverage. This is especially true if you're diagnosed with cancer.

The second thing you need to check is how good your insurance really is. See the section later in this chapter called How good is your health insurance policy? for help in deciding whether you have enough coverage.

Okay, if everything is in order, you're ready to make your first appointment.

---

7 important questions to ask your doctor

At this point, your doctor may be ready to make a diagnosis and recommend a treatment, or he may need to wait for some test results to come back. Depending on what he suspects may be your problem, he may order further tests or refer you to a urologist. In any case, this is a good time to ask him some questions, such as:

- Will these tests definitely diagnose my problem?

- What else could be causing my problem?

- What is the least-risky treatment? Is it an option for me?

- Why won't a certain treatment work for me?

- What are the risks associated with this treatment?

- How likely is it that this treatment will completely solve my problem?

- What are the risks of leaving the problem alone?

If your family doctor doesn't answer questions to your satisfaction or you feel he is uninformed, ask for a referral to a urologist. If your condition appears to be a complicated problem of the urinary/reproductive system or it doesn't improve after a few months, many family doctors will automatically refer you to a urologist. Keep in mind that you'll also want to ask these questions of any urologist you see.

Choosing the best urologist

Urologists have medical training in both surgery and urology. Because many men with prostate problems are first diagnosed by a family doctor, they find it both helpful and convenient to have the family doctor oversee their care under the urologist.

While you'll probably want to keep your family doctor's recommendation of a urologist in mind, there are some other factors you may want to consider. Often, choosing the best urologist depends on what condition you need treated.

Different urologists may have different levels of experience in treating the various disorders. Whether you're suffering from benign prostatic hyperplasia (BPH), impotence, or prostate cancer, your quality of care and your satisfaction with the treatment may depend on your willingness to shop around a little.

You may find some comfort in the fact that urologists are rarely accused of providing less than adequate care to their patients compared to other kinds of doctors. Nonetheless, you still need to be actively involved with your doctor's decisions to make sure you get the best-quality care.

You may want to ask your family doctor to take an especially active role in monitoring all medicines you take, including any supplements or herbal remedies. You also should keep a current list of any drugs, herbs, or supplements you take, and make sure each doctor you see gets a copy of your list. These precautions can help protect you from the most common cause of medical injury — drug complications.

At the urologist's office

Your first visit to the urologist will be similar to seeing your family doctor. He'll also want to know as much about your past medical history as possible, so bring copies of the urination diary, sexual history, and medical history that you prepared for your family doctor.

He may want to do repeat tests of the rectal and PSA exams. In addition, he may want you to undergo a number of other tests, depending on what he thinks your problem could be. For a complete description of these tests, see Chapter 14.

How to give your doctor a checkup

Whether you're looking for a general practitioner or a specialist, such as a urologist, it pays to check him out. The first place to start checking is the American Medical Association's Physician Masterfile. This is a computerized database that tracks licensed medical doctors from medical school to retirement.

This database will tell you where the doctor went to school, when he graduated, if he's certified in any specialties, if any disciplinary action has ever been taken against him, states he's licensed in, and when he was licensed. For information from Masterfile, call (312) 464-5000.

Another good source of information on disciplinary actions taken against doctors by state medical boards or the federal government is the Public Citizen Health Research Group. For more

> *It is a good idea to "shop around" before you settle on a*
> *doctor. Ask about the condition of his Mercedes. Ask about*
> *the condition of his mechanic. Don't be shy!*
> *After all, you're paying for it!*
> Dave Barry, American humorist

information, write to them at 2000 P Street N.W., Washington, DC 20036.

Since you're looking for a urologist, you may want to contact the American Board of Medical Specialties (ABMS) at (800) 776-2378. The reason? Almost 30 percent of the doctors who call themselves specialists haven't been certified by a board of medical specialties. A doctor who specializes in urology is referred to as a *Diplomate* of the American Board of Urology. Currently, there are only about 7,700 qualified practicing urologists in the United States.

In order to be board certified, a doctor must complete a specific training program and pass a very difficult exam. In addition to asking if a doctor is board certified, you may also want to ask the ABMS what year he was certified. Urologists who were certified before 1985 never have to seek recertification, although they may do it voluntarily. However, any urologist certified after 1985 does have to be recertified within 10 years. A urologist who gets recertified every 10 years whether he's required to or not may be more likely to keep up with the latest medical knowledge.

However, Dr. Timothy B. McCall, author of *Examining Your Doctor*, cautions that although credentials are important, they probably shouldn't be your sole criteria for choosing a doctor. According to him, "Good credentials increase the odds that a doctor is good, but they aren't as important as is commonly assumed."

Consider the following points when selecting a doctor. If your doctor is a specialist, the ABMS can answer many of these questions for you. If you belong to a health maintenance organization (HMO), the member services department should be able to give you this information.

▶ What hospitals is the doctor affiliated with? A doctor with no hospital affiliations could be a doctor to stay away from. It may mean his hospital privileges have been revoked and hospital officials are unsure of his qualifications. To find the very best doctor, look for a doctor on the attending staff of a prestigious hospital. But keep in mind that hospital reputations vary from specialty to specialty. A little-known hospital can sometimes have the best reputation in a certain field.

▶ Does your doctor serve on a medical school faculty? If he does and the school is reputable, this usually indicates a good treatment track record. You should still look for a doctor who is involved in direct patient care on a daily basis instead of spending most of his time in the classroom.

▶ Does your doctor keep up with the latest developments in urology? Take this book to the doctor with you. Ask about the newest treatments discussed in later chapters.

▶ Finally, feel free to ask your doctor any questions concerning his qualifications or your health. If he gets angry, impatient, or exasperated, get another doctor.

What to do when your doctor suggests surgery

If your doctor says surgery is the best way to handle your problem, don't panic, but do get a second opinion (and even a third if you feel like it). You should be especially careful to get a second opinion if your doctor seems close-minded to every option except surgery or isn't familiar with possible alternatives. (You'll read about those in later chapters.)

You may want to ask your doctor to recommend someone to give you a second opinion, or you may feel more comfortable finding someone on your own. Be sure you seek a second opinion from a doctor who is qualified to treat your condition.

If you let your doctor know you're planning to get a second opinion, you can request that your records be sent to the doctor giving the second opinion. You'll save both time and money by not having to undergo the same medical tests again.

Your right to your medical records

You may not know it and your doctor may not be inclined to tell you, but in many states you have a legal right to possess a copy of your medical records. Doctors and hospitals must give you, at your expense, all test results, diagnostic information, laboratory reports, X-rays, prescriptions, and any other medical information you ask for.

Not only do you often have the right to see your records, you should want to see them. Since your employer and your insurance company have access to them, you need to make sure they are accurate. An inaccuracy in your medical records may cause an insurance company to reject your claim someday.

Of course, even if you don't live in a state that gives you the legal right to your records, any doctor worth his degree will be eager to share your medical information with you. It's also a good idea to keep your own personal medical record at home.

Check with your insurer to see if they will pay for a second opinion. This is also a good time to find out if they will cover the cost of surgery.

If you're covered by Medicare (Part B, Medicare Supplementary Medical Insurance), it will pay for part of the cost of a second and even a third opinion as long as it is for a condition covered by Medicare. You'll have to meet your deductible and your copayment. However, you do not have to pay the deductible and copayment if Medicare's Peer Review Organization requires that you get a second opinion.

If you have Medicare insurance, call the Medicare carrier in your area for names of doctors who accept Medicare assignment. Accepting assignment means those doctors will charge no more for their second opinion or other services than the Medicare-approved amount. You will find the name of your carrier in *The Medicare Handbook*. If you need a copy of this book, contact your local Social Security office.

Talk your way to better health

It's been said that real men don't eat quiche, help with the housework, or make very good patients. While the first two may do you no more harm than making your wife mad (which may actually be pretty dangerous by itself), the last one can be very hazardous to your health.

That's according to a study by researchers at the Health Institute of the New England Medical Center in Boston. They found that during doctor visits men tend to be much more passive than women. That habit appears to add up to poorer health for men.

In an analysis of 296 people, including 115 men, researchers noted that men asked fewer questions and gave less information about themselves and how they were feeling than women did. In fact, in a typical 15-minute doctor visit, men didn't ask one question while women asked six.

However, if the man's doctor is a woman, he does seem to fare somewhat better. Not only do men give women doctors twice as much information as they give male doctors, they also generally report fewer problems from their illnesses.

Men, if you want better health with fewer complications, the solution is simple: Talk to your doctor and ask questions.

Best ways to choose a surgeon

One way to find a qualified surgeon is to review all the medical literature on the type of operation you will be having to see which doctors have written articles on that particular procedure. You can find this information in the *Index Medicus* at most medium-sized libraries, or you can do a computer search of the Medline database if you or your local library has access to this online medical library.

You will also want to make sure that any surgeon you choose is board-certified in his specialty. See the section earlier in this chapter called *How to give your doctor a checkup* for more information on board-certified doctors.

In addition, it's a good idea to find out if the hospital or outpatient center where the surgery will be performed is accredited by a nationally recognized organization, such as the Joint Commission on Accreditation of Healthcare Organizations (JCAHO) or the Accreditation Association for Ambulatory Health Care. Generally, hospitals that have gone to the trouble to be accredited offer higher quality care than hospitals that haven't. To find out if a hospital is accredited, contact your local or state hospital association.

14 questions you must ask before surgery

Since surgery of any sort is such a serious undertaking, you need to be sure you really need it. You also want to be sure your doctor is qualified and has plenty of experience. Here are some questions you should ask:

- Why do I need this surgery?

- What are my alternatives to surgery?

- What will happen if I don't have surgery?

- What are the risks of this procedure?

- How many surgeries of this type have you done?

- What is your success rate? Be sure to ask how the doctor defines a successful surgery. You may define a successful surgery for an enlarged prostate as one that completely relieves all your symptoms, while the doctor may define successful as one that relieves 90 percent of your symptoms. If you don't clear up your expectations before surgery, you may be very disappointed or downright mad afterward. It's a good idea to ask your doctor if any of his other patients who've had the same surgery you're considering would be willing to contact you. If they do, ask them how satisfied they were with their results.

- What, if any, side effects should I expect?

- Will this be the only surgery I'll need, or is it likely I'll need more operations?

- How long will I have to stay in the hospital?

- Will I need a catheter after surgery? If so, for how long?

- Will I need medicine after surgery?

- How long will I be out of work?

- How soon after surgery can I have sexual intercourse?

- Will any other activities, such as lifting heavy objects, be limited after surgery? If so, for how long? If you have particular sports or other hobby activities in mind, be sure to ask about those specifically.

You need to be satisfied with the answers to these questions and any others you have before you agree to give your informed consent for the surgery to proceed. If your doctor isn't willing to take time to answer your questions, find another doctor.

What those fancy titles really mean

Typically, on a doctor's nameplate, you'll find an astonishing array of letters following his name. Although they look quite impressive and impossible to decipher, they're not. Here are some handy hints to help you understand what all those letters really mean:

M.D. — Of course, this stands for medical doctor.

D.A.B.U. — Diplomate of the American Board of Urology

D.M.R.D. — Diploma in Medical Radio-Diagnosis

D.M.R.T. — Diploma in Medical Radio-Therapy

F.A.C.P. — Fellow of the American College of Physicians

F.A.C.S. — Fellow of the American College of Surgeons

F.I.C.S. — Fellow of the International College of Surgeons

F.R.C.P. — Fellow of the Royal College of Physicians

F.R.C.S. — Fellow of the Royal College of Surgeons

M.R.C.S. — Member of the Royal College of Surgeons

M.S. — Master of Science or Master of Surgery

P.A. — Professional Association. All this means is that the doctor is a member of a legally formed group practice.

P.C. — Professional Corporation. This means the same thing as P.A. The term P.C. is simply preferred in some states.

Any titles that indicate your doctor is a fellow or member indicates your doctor has paid dues to have a membership in those groups. Also, the term college does not mean the organization is affiliated with a college. It's simply a fancy name for an organization that probably offers some developmental courses and may sponsor an annual convention.

However, some of these organizations require their members to meet fairly strict professional standards. Many of these organizations also provide educational materials that help keep doctors up-to-date with the latest medical developments in their fields. For example, doctors who are members of the American Urological Association (AUA) stay on top of things through meetings, journals, bulletins, and newsletters the AUA sponsors.

Calculate the cost of surgery

Before you schedule any surgery, be sure to discuss the costs with your surgeon. Ask what his fees are, as well as those of his assistants. Keep in mind that you'll also be billed by everyone who assists in your surgery, such as the anesthesiologist and any medical consultants.

You'll also want to check the rates of the hospital where you'll be staying. Call the hospital business office for this information. To calculate the total amount, you'll need to know how many days you'll be staying in the hospital. Your doctor can usually tell you this.

Also, you may be able to save yourself money by asking your doctor if you are a candidate for outpatient surgery — generally a much cheaper option than surgery that requires a hospital stay.

Finally, find out how much of the bill your insurance will cover. If you cannot cover any remaining costs, tell your surgeon. You may be able to work out a mutually acceptable payment plan.

How do your doctor's costs compare?

Want to know how your doctor's costs compare with other doctors in your area without doing a lot of legwork or making a million phone calls?

For just a few bucks and only one phone call, you can find out. Simply call the Health Care Cost Hotline at (900) 225-2500. For $2 to $4 per minute, you'll learn the most commonly charged fee and range of fees nationwide for more than 7,000 medical procedures.

Handling insurance issues

Your type of insurance may affect your choice of doctor. For example, people covered by an HMO or Medicare often have fewer options than people with private insurance. Even if your choice is somewhat limited, that shouldn't stop you from asking questions about expertise and experience to help you choose the best doctor.

How good is your health insurance policy?

The first thing you need to check is the financial stability of your insurer. Insurance companies are rated financially by companies like A.M. Best, Standard & Poor's, Moody's, and Duff & Phelps. Make sure any company you buy life, health, or disability insurance from is rated A, A+, or AA. One of those ratings indicates the company is financially sound and will be able to pay your claims. Your insurance agent should be able to show you this rating in writing. If he can't, there's something wrong with either the company or the agent. Find a new company.

Next, look for gaps in what's covered. Read all the fine print to be sure you know exactly what your policy does and doesn't cover.

Look for a stop-loss amount. After you've spent a set amount on deductibles and copayments, does the company step in to pay or hang you out to dry? A bill for a complicated medical procedure

Report your results

Just like it's your doctor's duty to give you the best possible care he's capable of, it's your duty to let your doctor know how things turned out, especially if they go wrong.

Naturally, if you don't tell your doctor when things go wrong, he won't know. And, more likely than not, he'll assume things went right and note one more successful treatment (yours, he thinks) in his little black book.

Most people don't have a problem reporting difficulties that pop up soon after treatment. It's only after a couple of years have passed or when they've moved away and found a new doctor that they neglect to report new problems.

Whether your feedback is positive or negative, now or several years from now, let your doctor know. This information will help him determine how successful his treatments really are and help him improve them as needed.

Not only does this help ensure you'll get better care and satisfaction, it will help other people get the best possible treatment, too.

---

could leave you with a 20 percent copayment of more than $100,000 if there is no stop-loss amount in your policy. Keep in mind that your maximum out-of-pocket expense may be different for different treatments.

Note the cap on benefits. Example: Suppose your policy has a $500,000 lifetime cap. That leaves you responsible for any bills after that amount. Good policies will have at least a $1 million to $2 million cap.

If your policy has all of these features, hold on to it. If it doesn't, look for another plan. If you're on your employer's plan, then you have several options:

- Pass up your employer's plan and buy a good plan yourself.

- If you get to choose your fringe benefits, opt for others such as life insurance or disability and pay for your own health care.

- Supplement the employee plan. You may be able to pay more for better coverage under your employer's policy. If not, consider a major medical plan with a large deductible to cover catastrophes.

Get the most for your health insurance dollars

Insurance companies regularly deny claims and refuse to pay for the full cost of treatment. Don't let it happen to you. Here's how to squeeze every penny possible from your health insurance company:

Read your full contract. Your employer or insurer probably gave you a summary of your health insurance when you signed up. Get a copy of the full contract from your insurer, and slowly read the entire policy. Take notes, and ask your insurance agent or benefits manager to explain anything you don't understand. Important exclusions are often listed in the fine print and footnotes.

Know the limitations. If you know your insurance won't cover an extra day in the hospital, plan to go home a day earlier if possible.

Check in advance whether you're covered for something. The insurance company certainly isn't going to let you know when you should have filed a claim. If you're covered for something but don't know it, you may as well not be covered.

Pay premiums on time, by check only. One of the chief reasons insurers cite for canceling a policy or denying a claim is nonpayment of premiums. Send your payments directly to the insurer, not to your agent.

Get a doctor's prescription for every medical product or service you buy. This not only includes drugs and tests but also items you purchase for problems related to your prostate, such as incontinence or impotence. If you need adult diapers temporarily after prostate surgery, ask your doctor to write a prescription. Also, you should ask for a prescription for products designed to help you overcome impotence, such as vacuum pumps or penile implants.

Keep detailed records of all medical expenses. Write down the names of the doctors you saw, dates of visits, and what was done. Even include the cost of mileage to and from the doctor's office. If your insurance doesn't cover it, you may still be able to take it off your taxes.

Record all contact with your insurance company. If you've called to ask whether an expense is covered and you're told that it is, ask the person you spoke with to send you a response in writing. When you submit your claim, submit it to that person, reminding him of your conversation.

Photocopy everything. Never send a claim or any medical document to the insurer without photocopying it first.

Submit claims right away. Most policies have a 90-day deadline for submitting claims. (There's also a limit to how long the insurer can take to get back to you.)

Send in bills you know won't be covered. Some bills aren't covered, but do go toward your deductible. The insurer won't count them, though, if you don't send them in.

Use the "participating providers." Some plans give you a discount for using certain doctors and hospitals.

Ask your doctor for an itemized statement. Some medical care providers don't or can't give a second statement, so keep the original safely filed.

Find out if you need to file for major medical reimbursement, too. Don't just assume that one check is all you get. Sometimes you have to file separate claims for your basic plan and your major medical plan. You get reimbursed by your basic plan, then you file the balance under your major medical.

Submit to your primary carrier first. If you need to submit two claims (to two insurance companies or to a basic and a major medical plan), find out who you should send your claim to first. If you send them in the wrong order, you may not get paid.

Use the toll-free number. Calls to your insurance company can be expensive if you don't use the 800 number. Find out the best time to call so you won't have to wait.

Take a filled-out insurance form to the doctor's office. If you're going to a new doctor, this will speed up their claims-filing process. A few days later, check to make sure the office filed your claim.

Bunch as much medical care into one calendar year as possible. That will help you meet your deductible.

Try to get reimbursed for services that aren't covered. Call your insurer and ask if there are any circumstances under which the service would be covered. Sometimes a service is covered if you receive it at a hospital clinic instead of at your doctor's office.

Don't just accept it if your claim is denied or you think you haven't been paid enough. If you stick to it, you have a good chance of getting your claim approved or getting more money. Immediately submit a written request asking for information about the appeals process, the reason for the denial or decreased amount, and the kinds of information the insurer would require to reconsider your claim. Ask for a reply by a certain date.

Resubmit your claim. Include whatever medical information might counter their reason for denying your claim. Include copies of all previous correspondence, and tell them they can call your doctor or medical provider. Be sure to let your doctor know he may be contacted. Also, state that you will call a specific person on a specific date if you haven't received a reply within four weeks.

If you are wrongly denied again, contact the state insurance department. Send copies of all your correspondence with the insurance company to them, including a copy of your policy (with the related parts highlighted), and ask them to schedule a hearing on your case. Small claims court is another option.

Keep your doctor bills in line

It happens all the time. You turn over your doctor or hospital bill to the insurance company, and you get rejected. The insurance company says your medical bill exceeds the "customary" or "usual" charge, and they refuse to pay the full amount of the bill.

Don't complain to the insurance company yet. Your doctor may be overcharging you. Insurance companies decide how much they will pay for a medical service by taking an average of fees charged by doctors and hospitals within your zip code.

First, ask your doctor why he charged more. You can take your doctor's answer back to the insurance company and possibly convince them to give you more money.

Second, limit visits to doctors in nearby upscale neighborhoods. If you live in a small town, don't go to see a doctor in a big city unless you have a good reason to do so. Remember, the insurance reimbursement is based on an average fee in your zip code.

Finally, fight the battle before you go to the doctor. Unless you have a medical emergency, find out before you see the doctor how much he normally charges. Then call your insurance company and ask how much it will allow for that service. If your doctor's fees are too high, tell him so. He may be willing to lower his price. Or you may choose to visit another doctor.

Don't count too much on Uncle Sam

Even though you're eligible for Medicare coverage once you reach age 65, you can't count on it to take care of all your medical costs. You still have to pay deductibles, coinsurance, and charges for services Medicare doesn't cover.

You have three choices to keep your health care costs under control:

- You can stay on your employer's health insurance plan after you retire.

- You can buy Medigap insurance to fill in Medicare holes.

- You can enroll in an HMO that has a contract to serve people on Medicare.

Medicare has two parts. If you're eligible for Medicare, you're automatically enrolled in Part A at age 65. You're also automatically enrolled in part B at the same time unless you state that you don't want it. Here's what's covered and what's not under both parts:

Part A
For the first 60 days you are in the hospital, you'll pay $760 (1997 figures). Medicare pays the rest. After the first 60 days, the longer you stay in, the less Medicare pays.

Medicare will pay for your first 20 days in a skilled nursing facility. Neither Medicare nor Medigap insurance will pay for most nursing home care.

Medicare will pay for all of your home health care services and medical supplies you need at home, but it only pays 80 percent of medical equipment costs. You have to pay the other 20 percent.

Medicare pays most of the costs of hospice care for terminally ill people.

You pay for the first three pints of blood you receive. Medicare pays for the rest.

Part B
For a doctor's services, medical and surgical services and supplies, physical therapy and speech therapy, tests, and medical equipment — both in the hospital and out — Medicare pays

80 percent. You pay a $100 deductible plus the other 20 percent. You pay half of the charges for mental health services.

Medicare covers all the costs for blood or urine tests and other lab services.

As you can see, Medicare leaves plenty of gaps. Besides the $100 deductible and the 20 percent copayment, you pay for your own prescription drugs, for routine physicals, for your first three pints of blood, for full-time home nursing care, and for nursing home care. Also, Medicare only pays for a limited number of days in a hospital or skilled nursing facility.

If your retirement package didn't include health insurance and you don't want to join an HMO, you'll need to buy a Medigap policy. For a period of six months after you enroll in Medicare Part B, you have a guaranteed legal right to the Medigap policy of your choice regardless of your health conditions. During these six months, you can buy any Medigap policy sold by any insurer doing Medigap business in your state.

You also are entitled to a "free look" at any policy. This means the insurance company must give you at least 30 days to review a Medigap policy. If you decide you don't want it, you can send it back and have all your money refunded.

Finally, it's against the law for any Medigap insurance salesman to sell you a policy that duplicates coverage you already have. If you think at any point you've been a victim of a dishonest insurance company, call the federal toll-free number for filing insurance complaints — (800) 638-6833.

Avoid the cancer insurance scam

Cancer insurance is a rip-off, according to a congressional subcommittee that investigated it. Instead, buy a major medical policy with catastrophic coverage — that is, one with a high deductible of anywhere from $2,000 to $5,000. The premiums will be lower than a low-deductible policy, and you'll be covered for illnesses other than cancer as well.

How to choose the best Medigap insurance

All people over 65 and on Medicare need Medigap insurance. Medigap covers medical bills that government-provided health insurance doesn't pay. The federal government has set standards for 10 types of Medigap policies, called A through J. Insurance companies can sell the low-cost "core" policy plus any or all of the others.

Here are some pointers on choosing a policy:

▶ In comparing prices among policies, check the insurer's premium schedules, called outlines of coverage. Find out if the premiums will remain relatively stable or will rise each year as you age. You may be better off with a policy costing more initially than one that gets more expensive each year.

▶ Check for low-cost policies among social or professional organizations to which you belong or can join.

▶ Look for an insurer that offers electronic billing, which can save you money and irritation. Also, some insurers provide crossover billing — that means your Medicare bills go automatically to the Medigap insurance company.

Here is a list of the 10 standard plans and the benefits provided by each:

Plan A (the basic policy) consists of these basic benefits:

• Coverage for the Part A coinsurance amount ($190 per day in 1997) for the 61st through the 90th day of hospitalization in each Medicare benefit period.

• Coverage for the Part A coinsurance amount ($380 per day in 1997) for each of Medicare's 60 nonrenewable lifetime hospital inpatient reserve days used.

• After all Medicare hospital benefits are exhausted, coverage for 100 percent of the Medicare Part A eligible hospital expenses. Coverage is limited to a maximum of 365 days of additional inpatient hospital care during the policyholder's lifetime. This benefit is paid either at the rate Medicare pays hospitals under its Prospective Payment System (PPS) or under another appropriate standard of payment for hospitals not subject to the PPS.

- Coverage under Medicare Parts A and B for the reasonable cost of the first three pints of blood or equivalent quantities of packed red blood cells per calendar year unless replaced in accordance with federal regulations.

- Coverage for the coinsurance amount for Part B services (generally 20 percent of approved amount; 50 percent of approved charges for outpatient mental health services) after $100 annual deductible is met.

Plan B includes the basic benefits plus:

- Coverage for the Medicare Part A inpatient hospital deductible ($760 per benefit period in 1997).

Plan C includes the basic benefits plus:

- Coverage for the Medicare Part A deductible.

- Coverage for the skilled nursing facility care coinsurance amount ($95 per day for days 21 through 100 per benefit period in 1997).

- Coverage for the Medicare Part B deductible ($100 per calendar year in 1997).

- 80 percent coverage for medically necessary emergency care in a foreign country, after a $250 deductible.

Plan D includes the basic benefits plus:

- Coverage for the Medicare Part A deductible.

- Coverage for the skilled nursing facility care daily coinsurance amount.

- 80 percent coverage for medically necessary emergency care in a foreign country, after a $250 deductible.

- Coverage for at-home recovery. The at-home recovery benefit pays up to $1,600 per year for short-term, at-home assistance with activities of daily living (bathing, dressing, personal hygiene, etc.) for those recovering from an illness, injury, or surgery. There are various benefit requirements and limitations.

Plan E includes the basic benefits plus:

- Coverage for the Medicare Part A deductible.

- Coverage for the skilled nursing facility care daily coinsurance amount.

- 80 percent coverage for medically necessary emergency care in a foreign country, after a $250 deductible.

- Coverage for preventive medical care. The preventive medical care benefit pays up to $120 per year for such things as a physical examination, serum cholesterol screening, hearing test, diabetes screenings, and thyroid function test.

Plan F includes the basic benefits plus:

- Coverage for the Medicare Part A deductible.

The bottom line? Be informed

The more you know about your condition, the more likely you are to get the best medical care. And these days, it's easier than ever to access the information you need.

On June 26, 1997, The National Library of Medicine launched a new service on the Internet that provides all Americans with free access to Medline, the world's largest collection of medical information. This gives you the same access to scientific studies that doctors have. In addition, the new Internet site also provides a link to Healthfinder, a government-sponsored site that provides easy-to-understand health information directly to consumers.

If you have access to a computer linked with the Internet either at home or through a local library, be sure to check out the National Library of Medicine site. Their Internet address is: http://www.nlm.nih.gov.

- Coverage for the skilled nursing facility care daily coinsurance amount.

- Coverage for the Medicare Part B deductible.

- 80 percent coverage for medically necessary emergency care in a foreign country, after a $250 deductible.

- Coverage for 100 percent of Medicare Part B excess charges.*

Plan G includes the basic benefits plus:

- Coverage for the Medicare Part A deductible.

- Coverage for the skilled nursing facility care daily coinsurance amount.

- Coverage for 80 percent of Medicare Part B excess charges.*

- 80 percent coverage for medically necessary emergency care in a foreign country, after a $250 deductible.

- Coverage for at-home recovery (see Plan D).

Plan H includes the basic benefits plus:

- Coverage for the Medicare Part A deductible.

- Coverage for the skilled nursing facility care daily coinsurance amount.

- 80 percent coverage for medically necessary emergency care in a foreign country, after a $250 deductible.

- Coverage for 50 percent of the cost of prescription drugs up to a maximum annual benefit of $1,250 after the policyholder meets a $250 per year deductible (this is called the "basic" prescription drug benefit).

Plan I includes the basic benefits plus:

- Coverage for the Medicare Part A deductible.

- Coverage for the skilled nursing facility care daily coinsurance amount.

- Coverage for 100 percent of Medicare Part B excess charges.*

- Basic prescription drug coverage (see Plan H for description).

- 80 percent coverage for medically necessary emergency care in a foreign country, after a $250 deductible.

- Coverage for at-home recovery (see Plan D).

Plan J includes the basic benefits plus:

- Coverage for the Medicare Part A deductible.

- Coverage for the skilled nursing facility care daily coinsurance amount.

- Coverage for the Medicare Part B deductible.

- Coverage for 100 percent of Medicare Part B excess charges.*

- 80 percent coverage for medically necessary emergency care in a foreign country, after a $250 deductible.

- Coverage for preventive medical care (see Plan E).

- Coverage for at-home recovery (see Plan D).

- Coverage for 50 percent of the cost of prescription drugs up to a maximum annual benefit of $3,000 after the policyholder meets a $250 per year deductible (this is called the "extended" drug benefit).

* Plan pays a specified percentage of the difference between Medicare's approved amount for Part B services and the actual charges (up to the amount of charge limitations set by either Medicare or state law).

Make the most of Medicare

When you turn 65, you're automatically enrolled in Medicare if you've signed on for Social Security benefits. Although you can't count on Medicare to cover all your medical bills, you can make more of the benefits you do have with the following tips:

▶ Be sure any doctors or hospitals you use are Medicare certified. Also, if you chose to pay a little extra and be covered by Part B of the Medicare system, you need to make sure any laboratories your doctor uses for your blood work or other tests are also Medicare certified.

▶ Ask your doctor if he will provide his services to you "under assignment." This means the doctor will accept Medicare's reimbursement to him as full payment for his services without charging you any extra.

For a list of doctors who work under assignment, check your local Social Security office for *The Medicare Participating Physician/Supplier Directory.* If your doctor won't agree to work under assignment, you may still be able to negotiate a reduced rate with him.

Insurance injustice

Lately, controversy has raged over insurers' newest cost-cutting proposal, "Least Costly Alternative (LCA)."

Under this system, people may be forced to choose the cheapest treatment option — not the one that's necessarily best for them. For example, men with prostate cancer may be forced to choose castration to control their cancer instead of hormone drugs because castration is the cheaper choice.

The American Prostate Society encourages men to fight this new proposal by writing personal letters of protest to the President of the United States and to the Secretary of Health and Human Services.

When you don't have health insurance, you still have options

If you're diagnosed with a serious medical condition, such as cancer, and you don't have health insurance, getting insurance may seem like the impossible dream. While there's no denying that it will be more difficult, you do have a couple of options.

▶ Try to get into a group plan. If your work or some other organization you know of offers a group plan that doesn't screen for pre-existing conditions, like cancer, join as soon as you can.

▶ If you're 65 or older or disabled, apply for Medicare coverage during open enrollment. During this time, Medicare must accept everyone who applies regardless of any existing condition.

▶ If you have a limited income or are disabled, you may be eligible for Medicaid. If you're under 65 and don't have insurance, check out this option by contacting your local or state department of social services.

▶ Check on disability insurance, which pays you if you become disabled and can't work. You can find out if you are eligible by contacting your local Social Security office.

▶ If you're a veteran, look into benefits offered by the Veterans Administration. They have a number of hospitals across the country that offer care to veterans.

▶ Call your state department of insurance to find out if your state sells comprehensive health insurance. Some states provide this service to people who can't get coverage because of a serious medical condition.

▶ Contact local city and county agencies to see what medical services they offer for people in need who are not covered by private medical insurance.

▶ Ask your doctor if there are any clinical trials in your area that you could enroll in. These trials give doctors the opportunity to test new drugs and treatments and give people the opportunity to try them, usually for free. For more information on clinical trials, see Chapter 9.

Get your insurance company to pay for herbal remedies

For certain conditions that affect (most men might say afflict is a more accurate description) the prostate, such as prostatitis and BPH, herbal remedies may offer as much relief as a prescription drug or surgery. A growing number of doctors even prescribe them.

And prescribe is precisely the key word that prompts some insurance companies to pay for herbal remedies the same way they would a typical drug prescription. If your doctor is open-minded about herbal remedies, ask if he'd be willing to prescribe the ones helpful for your condition.

Not all insurance companies are advanced enough in their thinking to be willing to pay just yet. If they would consider this option, they'd realize most herbal remedies would cost them a lot less than traditional drugs. American Western Life is leading the way in this field.

If you're interested in using herbal remedies, ask your insurance company about their herbal payment policy. If they're not willing to pay, you may want to point out that cutting edge insurance companies like American Western Life are finding that this is one policy that offers such a savings to insurers it has the potential to pay for itself.

In summary

If you've been having painful ejaculation or urination or you've noticed a need to urinate more frequently than in the past, see your doctor. Most men choose their family doctors for that first appointment.

You can make diagnosing your problem quicker and easier if you prepare for your appointment. Take your urination diary, a list of symptoms, and your sexual and medical histories. Remember to write down any questions you want to ask.

Once your doctor makes a diagnosis, learn all you can about your condition. The more knowledge you have and the more involved you are in your health care, the more likely you are to receive the best treatment.

If you need a urologist later, it's often a good idea to have your family doctor oversee your treatment. You may want to ask your family doctor to take an especially active role in monitoring all medicines you take, including any supplements or herbal remedies. This precaution can help protect you from the most common cause of medical injury — drug complications.

Also, to ensure that you get the best possible care, choose your urologist carefully and be sure to check his credentials and experience.

If your doctor suggests surgery, always get a second opinion unless it's a medical emergency. Both Medicare and private insurers often pay for this. If you decide surgery is the best option for you, you'll want to run through all of the questions discussed in this chapter. The more you understand about the procedure, the more likely you are to be satisfied with the outcome.

It's a good idea to make sure your insurance is in effect before you make your first doctor's appointment. If your doctor diagnoses a prostate condition that may involve a long, drawn-out treatment or an expensive treatment, you need insurance to protect yourself financially.

It's also important to carefully examine the insurance you have, whether you're covered by a private insurer or through Medicare, so you can maximize your benefits. You want to be sure you have enough insurance to cover your health care needs. Finally, if you don't have insurance and you are diagnosed with a serious condition, you do have several options that may help you cover costs.

The bottom line in dealing with your doctor and handling insurance issues: be informed. The more you know about your doctor, your condition, your treatment, and your insurance, the more likely your treatment will work and the less likely you'll have any unpleasant surprises on the road back to good health.

Life is a perpetual instruction in cause and effect.
Ralph Waldo Emerson,
American essayist, philosopher, and poet

3

Common prostate problems

Your body's natural protection

Just like other parts of your body, your prostate has defenses to protect against bacterial invaders. If the prostate detects a possible attack, it will pull out its heavy artillery in the form of white blood cells and natural antibodies. Zinc and certain amino acids also pack a powerful punch against bad bacteria.

Your body works hard to protect your prostate against bad bacteria and with good reason. Your prostate is located and designed in such a way that once the bad guys get in, it's very hard to get them out.

Identify your prostate problem

Generally, when it comes to prostate problems, symptoms fall into one of two categories — either irritative or obstructive.

To find out what kind of symptoms are bothering you, take the following test. Simply place a check by any symptom you have. Once you can classify your symptoms as irritative or obstructive, you'll have a better idea of whether it's an enlarged prostate or an infection that's causing your problems. Of course, you'll still need to see your doctor for a professional diagnosis and treatment.

- Do you urinate more frequently than in the past? (irritative) __yes __no

- Do you feel an urgent need to urinate? (irritative) __yes __no

- Is urinating painful? (irritative) __yes __no

- Do you often urinate only small amounts? (irritative)__yes __no

- Do you wake up at night to urinate? (irritative/obstructive) __yes __no

- Is pain in your bladder relieved by urinating? (obstructive) __yes __no

- Do you have problems completely emptying your bladder? (obstructive) __yes __no

- Do you have difficulty getting your urine stream started? (obstructive) __yes __no

- Has your urine stream decreased? (obstructive) __yes __no

Now, look back at your check marks. Add up how many you marked for obstructive symptoms and how many for irritative.

If most of your symptoms are irritative, you probably have an infection. If you have nearly equal amounts of both irritative and obstructive symptoms, you're likely suffering from an enlarged prostate. Inflammation usually causes frequency, urgency, pain, and burning.

Run down the list of symptoms listed at the beginning of different sections in this chapter. They may help you pinpoint just what your problem is.

Infection detection

If your symptoms are mostly irritative, this section is a good place to start looking for the root of your problem. If none of these conditions seem to be the cause of your problem, move to the section on benign prostatic hyperplasia (BPH). Many men with BPH have only irritative symptoms.

If you have both irritative and obstructive symptoms, browse through all the sections to see if one condition seems to apply to you more than the others. You still need to see a doctor for a formal diagnosis. However, if you know a little about the condition you're likely to have, you'll be in a better position to discuss your treatment options.

Prostate terms you need to know

Puzzled over the difference between prostatitis, prostatosis, prostatodynia, and a whole host of different "P" words you've heard describe prostate problems? Don't worry. You're not alone. Even doctors can't always agree on what to call certain disorders. To help you out, here's a brief rundown of what all those different "P" words mean.

Prostatitis – An inflamed prostate gland, which may or may not be infected.

Women can have prostate problems, too

No doubt any woman you know will deny it to her dying day, but women can have prostate problems, too.

Women have glands near the urethra called the paraurethral glands, which are very similar to the man's prostate. Just like the prostate, these glands can become inflamed and infected and even develop cancer. Plus, these glands also produce prostate specific antigen (PSA), although the levels are so small they can't be detected by blood tests like they can in men.

The treatment for this problem is similar to prostatitis treatment — a prescription of antibiotics, often for several weeks or more. Sitz baths can help relieve pain and irritation. Just like prostatitis, a paraurethral infection tends to recur.

If any woman you care about complains of a long-standing case of urethral syndrome (a catch-all diagnosis many doctors use when they can't determine what is causing the woman's continued urinary problems), tell her to ask her doctor about a possible problem with her paraurethral glands.

Prostatism – Any prostate problem that interferes with urine flow from the bladder. Traditionally, all lower urinary tract symptoms in older men were called prostatism.

Prostatodynia – A painful prostate with no apparent signs of inflammation or infection.

Prostatosis – Any problem with the prostate that isn't cancer or an inflammatory condition. This term is often used interchangeably with the term noninfectious prostatitis. Some doctors prefer prostatosis over nonbacterial prostatitis because of the possibility that bacteria may one day be linked to nonbacterial prostatitis.

Prostatic – Having to do with the prostate gland. For example, benign prostatic hyperplasia means an enlarged prostate.

Prostatalgia – Another term for prostatodynia.

Prostatomegaly – Enlargement of the prostate gland.

Pelvic pain syndrome – According to the National Institutes of Health's new classification of prostatitis, chronic pelvic pain syndrome is a combination of what were previously the separate categories of nonbacterial prostatitis and prostatodynia.

New prostate groupings aid diagnosis

In an attempt to find better ways of treating the irritating problem of prostatitis, researchers have recently reclassified the common categories of prostatitis. They hope the new classification system will allow doctors to more accurately diagnose and effectively treat prostatitis.

In the past, prostatitis had been classified into the following four groups:

- Acute bacterial prostatitis — Infection plus inflammation in the prostate. Generally responds quickly to antibiotics.
- Chronic bacterial prostatitis — Infection plus inflammation in the prostate. Although antibiotics can help, it usually takes much longer to clear up this infection than acute bacterial prostatitis.
- Nonbacterial prostatitis — Inflammation but no readily apparent sign of infection. May or may not respond to antibiotics.

- Prostatodynia — Prostate pain with no sign of either infection or inflammation. A few cases respond well to antibiotics. Researchers speculate prostatodynia may be caused by spasms of the bladder, pelvic, or rectal muscles.

Working with the National Institutes of Health, researchers have come up with a new classification system they hope will allow them to more accurately identify and treat each case of prostatitis. Here's a brief look at the new classification system:

I. Acute bacterial prostatitis — A rare condition that involves infection plus inflammation. Generally responds quickly to antibiotics.

II. Chronic bacterial prostatitis — A fairly rare condition that involves infection plus inflammation. Traditionally more difficult to treat than acute bacterial prostatitis.

III. Chronic pelvic pain syndrome — This is the new term for nonbacterial prostatitis and prostatodynia. It is divided into two parts:

IIIa. Inflammation is present in the prostate although there is no readily apparent sign of infection. This is what used to be called nonbacterial prostatitis.

IIIb. There is no sign of either infection or inflammation in the prostate. This is what used to be called prostatodynia.

IV. Asymptomatic prostatitis — This is a new category in the classification of prostatitis. This type of prostatitis causes no symptoms. It is often diagnosed during a test for prostate cancer.

Keep in mind that it will probably take some time before the new classification system becomes widely used. However, it will be useful for you to know both the old and the new way of classifying prostatitis so you can discuss your treatment options knowledgeably with your doctor.

9 steps to clear up urethritis

Watery discharge from penis
Opening of penis appears "glued" shut
Brownish or yellowish stain on the front of underwear
Itchy feeling inside penis

Feeling of discomfort in penis during urination

Any of these symptoms suggest urethritis, which is an inflammation of the urethra, the tube that carries urine from the bladder to the penis and out of the body. It may be caused by an infection, an irritation, or a minor injury.

See your doctor if you have an infection so he can prescribe antibiotics. Although untreated urethritis may eventually go away on its own, it can leave you with a worse problem — a urethral stricture or blockage. An injury or untreated infection can cause scar tissue to build up in the urethra. A urethral stricture occurs when this scar tissue shrinks, causing the urethra to narrow and sometimes even become shorter. This makes it difficult and painful to urinate or ejaculate. There is no natural remedy for a urethral stricture.

Generally, antibiotics will relieve your symptoms within 24 hours. However, to completely wipe out the infection, be sure to finish up all antibiotics no matter how soon you feel better.

Typically, urethritis is caused by an infection you picked up from your mate during sexual intercourse. These infections can be passed back and forth between partners, so it's a good idea to have your mate treated at the same time you are.

Here are some self-help suggestions to comfort and heal an irritated urethra:

When insomnia may mean BPH

If you've been irritated by interruptions to your sleep lately, your problem may be your prostate, especially if you typically make several trips to the bathroom each night. Feeling tired or being unable to go back to sleep after yet another trip to the john is often one of the first signs of BPH. See your doctor about treating your BPH and you'll likely solve your sleep problems at the same time.

▶ Soak in a sitz bath. Although sitz baths sound somewhat mysterious, they're really not. Sitz is simply a German word for seat. So, a sitz bath basically involves sitting for 15 minutes in a few inches of hot water. Sitz baths are soothing because they help relieve the discomfort of an irritated prostate. They also appear to improve circulation and healing.

▶ Don't squeeze on your penis to see if the discharge is still present. It's okay to inspect it gently.

▶ Clean your genitals and surrounding areas with plain, unscented soap.

▶ Say no to sex or use a condom until you're free of symptoms for two weeks.

▶ Drink eight glasses of water a day.

▶ Chug some cranberry juice. This will acidify your urine and possibly help prevent future problems. Also, some drugs work better if your urine is acidic.

In addition, modifying your sexual habits can help prevent future infections:

▶ Use the bathroom within 15 minutes after sex. It may help if you drink a glass of water before sex.

▶ Use latex condoms.

▶ If you use lubricants, make sure you use a water-soluble one, such as K-Y Lubricating Jelly.

The good news about benign prostatic hyperplasia (BPH)

Difficulty getting urine stream to start; also called hesitancy
Weak urine stream
Feeling of incomplete emptying after urination
Frequent need to urinate

Have to get up one or more times during the night to urinate
Dribbling, incontinence

Your symptoms suggest benign (noncancerous) prostate enlargement. This common condition affects up to 50 percent of all men by the time they reach 80 years. Autopsies suggest up to 80 percent of men may actually have BPH.

The good news is that only about half of the men with BPH need treatment. For men who do need relief, there are a number of effective treatments. Turn to Chapter 4 for an in-depth discussion of this common prostate problem.

Clear up confusion about prostatitis

If you've ruled out urethritis and BPH, that leaves prostatitis or prostatodynia as possible causes of your problem. Prostatitis appears to be a pretty common problem. Researchers estimate that about one out of every four men with a urinary problem has prostatitis.

Prostatitis is a general term that includes infections, inflammation, and nonbacterial conditions of the prostate. Literally, the word means "inflammation of the prostate." There are actually three different types of prostatitis: acute bacterial prostatitis, chronic bacterial prostatitis, and chronic nonbacterial prostatitis. Although prostatodynia is not technically a type of prostatitis, it is often lumped together with different types of prostatitis.

Determining what kind of prostatitis you have can be a real trick even for your doctor. Your doctor bases his diagnosis on whether you have an inflammation or an infection in your prostate. An infection is caused by bacteria. An inflammation is caused by something other than bacteria. It's easy to confuse and even misuse the two words because the symptoms of an infection or inflammation can be exactly alike. It will help if you remember that infection rarely occurs without inflammation, but inflammation often occurs without infection.

How to beat acute bacterial prostatitis

Fever, chills, flu-like symptoms

Drug danger: BPH and cold cures don't mix

If you have BPH or prostatitis, watch out for cold remedies like decongestants and antihistamines. Some of these products contain ingredients that can interfere with urine flow. To protect yourself from potential problems, be sure to always tell your doctor what medicines you take, both prescribed and over-the-counter.

In addition, when buying decongestants or antihistamines, always check the label. Products that could cause problems for men with BPH or prostatitis often carry a small warning in fine print.

Blood in the urine
Pain in the lower back and perineum (the area between the
    scrotum and anus)
Extremely painful and/or urgent urination
Total inability to urinate (sometimes)

Typically, symptoms of acute bacterial prostatitis come on so quickly, so furiously, and so painfully they're frightening. That's your body's way of urgently warning you that you need to see a doctor NOW! If your condition has reached a critical point, you may need to stay in the hospital a few days. In fact, a case of untreated acute bacterial prostatitis can eventually lead to an abscess that has to be drained surgically because it will no longer respond to antibiotics.

The good news is that acute bacterial prostatitis is one of the most easily treated prostate problems. Antibiotics often wipe out the infection completely, and many times it never returns. Most experts recommend a four- to six-week course of antibiotics. This will help completely eliminate the infection and reduce the risk of your infection becoming chronic.

Acute bacterial prostatitis is most commonly caused by a bacterial infection. Infected urine may be responsible for transmitting the bacteria.

When your doctor checks your prostate with a digital rectal exam, he will find it soft and boggy, and you will find it very, very painful.

The best way to test for this problem is with a simple urine culture. If the culture is positive for bacteria, antibiotics will normally clear up the problem fairly quickly.

In addition to taking your antibiotics exactly as your doctor prescribed them, there are some other things you can do to speed your recovery:

▶ Rest in bed.

▶ Drink lots of water.

▶ Say no to sex until your condition improves.

▶ Use a stool softener. Because the rectum is right behind the prostate, straining to have a bowel movement could make your already tender prostate ache even more. A stool softener will help prevent that.

4 ways to combat chronic bacterial prostatitis (CBP)

Frequent urinary urgency
Need to urinate frequently
Painful urination
Pain in lower back or lower section of the stomach area
Feeling of heaviness or pressure behind the scrotum
Painful ejaculation
Symptoms may come and go

Chronic bacterial prostatitis may follow a case of acute prostatitis that wasn't completely cured. This condition also appears to be linked with repeated urinary tract infections (UTIs). In fact, unless you've had a case of untreated acute prostatitis or have had a urinary tract infection diagnosed by a doctor in the past, it's unlikely that you have chronic bacterial prostatitis.

A short-term course of antibiotics usually won't clear up a case of chronic bacterial prostatitis. It usually takes 10 to 12 weeks of full-strength antibiotics to knock out the infection. Because it's difficult for antibiotics to penetrate the prostate, many doctors also

Montezuma's revenge linked to chronic prostate infections

The same family of bacteria responsible for Montezuma's revenge (also called traveler's diarrhea), as well as those deadly hamburger disasters in the Northwest in the early 1990s, also appears to be responsible for most of the cases of bacterial prostatitis.

Of the 5 to 10 percent of men who actually have chronic bacterial prostatitis, most of those cases can be linked to that most bothersome family of bacteria — Escherichia coli. Most cases of acute bacterial prostatitis are also caused by E. coli.

Although E. coli normally lives in the intestines without causing any problems, it can cause severe illness if it moves to other areas of the body. Usually, different varieties of the bacteria are responsible for causing food poisoning and prostatitis.

recommend a maintenance course of antibiotics for several more months to completely eliminate the infection.

In addition to antibiotics, here are some other tips for dealing with chronic bacterial prostatitis:

▶ Avoid alcohol.

▶ Stay away from spicy foods.

▶ Relieve pain by sitting in a few inches of hot water for 15 minutes twice a day. This is called a "sitz bath."

▶ Ejaculate regularly. Some experts say regular ejaculation, either through sexual intercourse or masturbation, is important because it routinely empties the glands and ducts of the prostate so an infection is less likely to maintain its hold there. If you object to masturbation for any reason, ask your urologist about prostate massage. He can either do this for you or show you or your mate how to do it.

Prostate stones, similar to stones found in the gallbladder or kidneys, are one of the main causes of a prostate infection that fails to respond to treatment. Prostate stones are normally harmless unless they harbor bacteria. Then, they serve as a breeding ground for repeated infections. Also, they often don't allow antibiotics to work properly. If your case is caused by prostate

Are antibiotics your best bet?

For some doctors, the symptoms of any type of prostatitis call for an automatic antibiotic prescription.

Before you accept one of these prescriptions and head for the nearest drugstore, consider this fact: The vast majority (90 to 95 percent) of men have nonbacterial prostatitis.

Does that mean antibiotics won't work? Well, it depends on which doctor you talk to. Some more traditional doctors may shun antibiotics, saying they can't treat a problem that wasn't caused by some sort of bacteria in the first place.

Other doctors, however, will want you to try a trial run of antibiotics to see if you show any improvement. That's because the latest line of thinking about nonbacterial prostatitis and prostatodynia is that they are caused by multiple bacteria or by bacteria that has yet to be identified, which is why it's not recognized during laboratory testing.

So, what should you do? Only you can decide, but you might consider trying nonantibiotic remedies first to see if they offer any relief before you bombard your body with heavy doses of antibiotics.

However, if home remedies don't help, by all means consider trying antibiotics. Many men have found antibiotics effectively relieved their so-called nonbacterial prostatitis or prostatodynia. In fact, about 40 percent of the men who have symptoms that point to prostatitis improve after a course of antibiotics.

stones that stubbornly refuse to respond to antibiotics, you may need surgery.

Knock out nonbacterial prostatitis (NBP)

Pain in the perineum, the area between the scrotum and anus
Pain in the genital area
Painful urination
Urgent and/or frequent need to urinate
Painful ejaculation

This is the most common type of prostatitis, occurring about eight times more often than any other kind. So far, researchers haven't been able to identify any bacteria that could be causing the problem, which is why this condition is referred to as nonbacterial prostatitis. Researchers speculate that uncommon bacteria, which haven't been identified, could be the culprits. Nonbacterial prostatitis has also been linked to jobs that involve a lot of sitting.

However, a recent study at the University of Washington revealed that difficult-to-detect bacteria may actually be the cause of 87 percent of the cases of chronic nonbacterial prostatitis. Seventy-seven percent of those cases involved bacteria that have never before been discovered or identified in laboratory testing. This would help explain why those so-called cases of "nonbacterial" prostatitis often respond so well to antibiotics.

Interestingly enough, all of the men selected for this study passed tests like the Meares-Stamey test, which has been the gold standard for the last 25 years in identifying bacterial prostatitis. See Chapter 14 *Diagnostic tests* for a complete description of the Meares-Stamey test as well as other tests used to diagnose prostate problems.

Until doctors definitely determine a cause and a reliable treatment for nonbacterial prostatitis, here are some simple, self-help suggestions to speed your recovery from prostatitis and prevent its recurrence:

Drink plenty of water. Increase your fluid intake to at least eight cups of water a day. This will help prevent a kidney infection.

Avoid jarring motions and prolonged sitting.

Exercise. Keep up your fitness program, but don't ride a bike. It could cause irritation. Walking is a good alternative.

Zap prostatitis with zinc. Pumpkin seeds contain lots of healing nutrients for your prostate, especially zinc and magnesium. Chicken livers, oysters, and dark turkey meat are also good sources of zinc.

Cut your chance of infection with vitamin C. Vitamin C is well known for its abilities to bolster your immune system, which may help your body fight off prostate infections more effectively. Good natural sources of vitamin C include orange juice, sweet red and green peppers, cantaloupe, brussels sprouts, and strawberries.

Ejaculate regularly. Some experts suggest that regular ejaculation is important for helping the prostate drain completely, which is vital for keeping infectious organisms at bay. So what's regular? Some doctors say as often as every other day, while others claim that once a week is plenty. Within those bounds, do whatever seems to work best for you.

Soothe your prostate with a sitz bath. Three times a day, sit in a tub of 6 to 8 inches of warm water for 15 minutes. A whirlpool bath is also helpful.

Try prostatic massage. Although it's best to get a doctor to do this for you, or at least demonstrate the proper technique the first time, you can do this yourself or get your mate to do it for you. If you don't have long enough arms to reach your rectum or long enough fingers to reach your prostate, you won't be able to do this procedure by yourself.

You'll need to make sure you have KY jelly and disposable gloves (nonlatex if you have a latex allergy) on hand before you begin. In addition, it's a good idea to keep some paper towels nearby to catch any discharge from your penis. You may also want to take a hot bath beforehand. This tends to make the massage more productive.

To begin, lie down and bring your hand around your body to your back, instead of trying to reach through your legs, to get in position. Gently insert a lubricated finger into your rectum. About an inch and a half in, you should feel a bump. That's your prostate. It may feel bigger than a walnut to you, especially if it's swollen. Also, you may or may not be able to feel a depression in the middle of it. That depends on how infected it is.

Firmly rub the prostate from side to side. Try to use slow, continuous pressure. You'll know you're doing it right if you feel a slight stinging or burning.

Massage may be pretty painful, depending on how swollen your prostate is. If you generally find this process painful, try taking some ibuprofen about an hour beforehand. Always urinate immediately after the massage to get rid of any bacteria that may have gotten into your urinary tract.

Some experts suggest daily massage, while others recommend a couple of times a week. Go with whatever schedule seems to give you the most relief.

Massage helps drain the prostate and may also increase blood flow to it. The main reason the prostate has difficulty fighting off infections is that the ducts in the prostate become blocked with inflamed debris. The prostate also has a limited blood supply, making it difficult for your immune system to properly defend your prostate from invaders. In addition, the poor blood supply makes it difficult for antibiotics to reach the prostate.

Eat a low-fat diet. A diet high in fat and cholesterol is particularly unhealthy for your prostate.

Simple step protects you and your mate

Several studies have identified sexually transmitted organisms, including Mycoplasma genitalium, Chlamydia trachomatis, Trichomonas, and Ureaplasma urealyticum, that may be responsible for causing prostatitis. If your doctor finds that your prostatitis is caused by a sexually transmitted organism, you may want to have your mate tested. If she's positive for the organism, it's a good idea for both of you to be treated at the same time. In the meantime, use condoms when engaging in sex.

If your doctor doesn't find any sexually transmitted organisms, but you suspect them as a possible cause, it's still a good idea to use condoms until you're sure any problems are cleared up in both you and your mate.

Avoid irritants in your diet. Alcohol, coffee, spicy foods, chocolate, and tomato products may irritate your prostate and possibly trigger spasms that can cause urine to backwash into your prostate, irritating it further.

Strike out stress and ax anxiety. Just as they seem to do in every other health problem, stress and anxiety may also aggravate prostatitis. Dr. Walt Stoll suggests that stress can cause unconscious tensing of the rectal muscles that may eventually lead to prostatitis by interfering with the blood flow both to and from the prostate.

Select soy. Preliminary animal studies suggest soy foods may help protect the prostate against inflammation. When rats were deprived of soy for 11 weeks, they developed severe prostate inflammations. Soy appears to block the testosterone production associated with prostatitis. Although researchers can't say for sure whether soy has the same effect on men, it won't hurt to add

---

For more information ...

When it comes to dealing with prostatitis, a disorder most doctors readily admit they don't have a good grasp on, the more you know, the better your chance of finding relief.

One of the best sources of easily understood information is the Prostatitis Foundation. Formed by a group of men frustrated by their own prostate treatments, the organization's goal is to increase awareness of the disease and provide information to men who are dealing with prostatitis. They also provide access to a phone bank of men with prostatitis who understand what you're going through and can offer helpful advice.

They could also refer you to a doctor who's willing to work with you, unlike those doctors whose own lack of understanding of the disorder makes them more likely to give you the brush off if you fail to improve with antibiotics.

You can write to them for more information at the Prostatitis Foundation Information Distribution Center, 2029 Ireland Grove Road, Bloomington, IL 61704. If you have Internet access, visit their site at http://www.prostate.org.

soy foods to your diet, and it may actually help prevent painful infections in the future.

Run for the rye — rye grass pollen extract, that is. Swedish Professor Eric Ask-Upmark found rye grass pollen extract (Secale cereale) to be helpful for chronic nonbacterial prostatitis over 30 years ago. Recent studies confirm his finding. Between 75 and 90 percent of men who take rye grass pollen extract either notice complete improvement or at least a considerable decrease in symptoms.

Rye grass pollen appears to be able to relieve some of the more difficult-to-treat symptoms of prostatitis, including painful and frequent urination as well as testicular pain, groin pain, perineal pain, and painful ejaculation.

Researchers aren't exactly sure how rye grass pollen works, although they suspect it may relieve the swelling associated with inflammation and help clear out clogged ducts in your prostate, which may harbor bacteria.

You can find the capsule form of rye grass pollen extract at most herb shops. Follow the dosage recommendations of the manufacturer. It may take at least three months before you notice a definite benefit. Some research suggests rye grass pollen may be helpful for prostatodynia as well.

Many of the rye grass pollen studies have been done using a product called Cernilton. If you'd prefer that brand over others, you can buy Cernilton from Cernitin America at (800) 831-9505.

Put pygeum to the test. The bark of the *pygeum africanum* tree, which grows in Africa, is used to make an extract for treating BPH and prostatitis. For relief of symptoms, some experts recommend taking 100 to 200 mg of pygeum per day. As an added benefit, some researchers think it may improve sexual performance.

If natural remedies don't work for you, ask your doctor about antibiotics. Almost half the men diagnosed with nonbacterial prostatitis find that antibiotics help. Other prescription options to consider include nonsteroidal anti-inflammatory drugs (NSAIDs) or alpha blockers. These drugs work by reducing inflammation and relaxing the muscles of the prostate gland.

Some men have even found relief with a short course of steroids. Several researchers have suggested that nonbacterial prostatitis may be caused by an auto-immune reaction. This means that for some reason, certain men with prostatitis have immune cells that attack their own prostates. This also happens in other diseases, such as some types of arthritis. When the researchers put these men on a short course of steroids, which suppress the immune system, symptoms seemed to improve.

Using herbal remedies wisely

Although herbs can give you more control over your health care, you should also use extra caution to stay safe. That's because herb quality and potency are not regulated by the Food and Drug Administration.

▶ Learn as much as you can about the herbs you plan to take. The American Botanical Council has published English translations of excellent German reports on herbs. They combine historical and traditional uses with modern scientific information.

▶ Buy herbs with the word "standardized" on the label. That means the manufacturer has tried to get a consistent amount of the healing herb in each pill.

▶ Don't use more of an herb than experts recommend. You may even want to use lower than normal doses, especially if you are older.

▶ Pay attention to your body's reaction to the herbs you take. Know the symptoms of toxicity and allergic reaction.

▶ Tell your doctor you are using herbs, especially if you also take prescription drugs.

Steer clear of prostatodynia

Lower back pain
Pain in pelvic and genital areas

Prostatodynia, which means "painful prostate," is often the term doctors use when they can't find any evidence of infection or inflammation in your prostate. Although the pain appears to be related to

Sitting pretty

Prostatitis not only puts a pinch on your prostate, it can make sitting a real pain in the butt. Some men say doughnut cushions sold at drugstores (originally designed for people suffering from hemorrhoids) can make sitting much more comfortable. Surprisingly, other men say sitting in a hard chair gives them the most relief.

the prostate, it may actually be caused by bladder, pelvic, or rectal muscles that are overly tense or generally out of whack.

Although most doctors don't associate prostatodynia with an infection, at least one study has found that men with prostatodynia were harboring bacteria in their prostates. Antibiotics were able to wipe out the infections.

Although there are some specific lifestyle changes you can make to relieve your prostatodynia, most of the self-help suggestions discussed in the nonbacterial prostatitis section also help with prostatodynia. In addition to those, here are two other tips:

► Stop stress. Most cases of prostatodynia occur in stressed-out men between the ages of 20 and 50 years.

► Can the caffeine. It will worsen spasms of your bladder, pelvic, or rectal muscles, which many researchers think are the cause of prostatodynia.

Other natural therapies you may want to try include relaxation exercises, massage, meditation, and biofeedback. Biofeedback lets you learn how to recognize changes in your body and use your mental powers to control those changes. You'll need the help of a trained biofeedback specialist and the right equipment to learn to control your brain waves. If your doctor is not trained in biofeedback, ask him if he can recommend someone who is.

If nothing else seems to help, ask your doctor about muscle relaxants, NSAIDs, and alpha blockers. These drugs can help relieve the bladder, pelvic, and rectal muscle spasms that may contribute to your prostatodynia. You may also want to ask your doctor about antibiotics.

The Filipino fix

Why have several hundred men with prostatitis flocked to Dr. Antonio Espinosa Feliciano's clinic in the Philippines?

Desperate for relief, they wanted to check out the claims of men who say they've been cured by Dr. Feliciano.

Feliciano's technique involves correctly identifying the offending bacteria and prescribing the appropriate antibiotic. Then, he has the man come into his office every other day for a prostate massage.

According to Feliciano, massage works like ejaculation in clearing out prostate secretions that may be clogging up the gland, which can contribute to and prolong prostate infections. However, Feliciano feels that massage does a more thorough job than ejaculation of clearing bothersome bacteria from the prostate. Massage also increases blood flow to the prostate, which improves the chance that antibiotics will be able to get into the prostate and be more effective.

Currently, researchers are attempting to validate Feliciano's method. According to J. Curtis Nickel, M.D., professor of urology at Queens University in Ontario, about 33 percent of the men who go to Feliciano and try his technique experience a significant improvement. Most of those men have suffered from nonbacterial prostatitis for years.

He notes that the men most likely to benefit have had prostatitis for less than a year. Dr. Nickel and his colleagues average a 50 percent cure rate among men they've treated using the Feliciano technique.

Man to man: words of wisdom from men with prostatitis

Men suffering from prostate problems, especially prostatitis, can find significant relief from prostate pain by making some simple lifestyle changes. Since everyone is different, your best bet is to try them all to determine which ones help you the most.

Drink lots of water, at least eight glasses every day. Although drinking less water may seem a more sensible choice (to avoid those frequent and urgent needs to urinate), you need plenty of water in your system to keep your urine from becoming too concentrated, which could cause a bladder infection or lead to dehydration.

Ease your pain with exercise. Some men find that walking regularly seems to help.

Control constipation. Hard bowel movements can put painful pressure on the prostate. Eating plenty of fiber can help prevent constipation. Add about 10 grams of fiber to your diet a day until you regularly eat 20 to 35 grams every day. Take care to introduce extra fiber into your diet gradually. Adding too much fiber too quickly could cause more constipation, gas, and bloating. Good sources of fiber, which means more than 6 grams of fiber per serving, include whole-wheat bread, beans, vegetables, fruits, and high-fiber cereals.

Put your prostate on ice. If a heating pad doesn't relieve your prostate pain, try ice. Some doctors suggest placing an ice cube in water until the rough edges melt off and it becomes smaller and then inserting the ice cube into the rectum. Supposedly, some men experience hours of pain relief this way.

Turn up the heat to knock out prostate problems

A technique called transurethral microwave thermotherapy (TUMT) may be the key to putting your prostate problems to rest for a while. TUMT involves sending computer-regulated microwave heat through a catheter to selected portions of the prostate.

Typically, TUMT has been used to destroy excess prostate tissue in men suffering with BPH. Recently, however, researchers have been investigating its ability to treat men whose prostatitis and prostatodynia have been unresponsive to traditional treatments.

Several studies have found TUMT to be a safe, effective, and long-lasting alternative to other treatments for prostatitis. In fact, one study that compared TUMT with a fake treatment found that 70 percent of the men receiving TUMT experienced significant improvement in their symptoms. Another study reported that improvement with TUMT therapy appeared to peak around three to six months after treatment with about 80 percent of the men reporting significant improvement. The benefits last for at least two years.

Allopurinol may ace prostatitis

Researchers have noted a number of possible causes for non-bacterial prostatitis, including bacteria, prostate stones, and psychological problems. Some researchers have also suggested that urine backflow into the prostate may even be the primary cause of most bacterial and nonbacterial cases of prostatitis.

The theory is that the backflow of urine may irritate the prostate and cause inflammation due to the build up of uric acid in the prostate ducts. To determine if their theory was valid, researchers decided to test allopurinol on men with prostatitis. Allopurinol is a drug commonly used to treat uric acid buildup in people with gout or kidney stones.

Researchers found allopurinol gave the men significant relief. It appears to work by reducing the concentration of uric acid in urine, which adds up to less irritation for the prostate. They concluded that allopurinol was a safe, effective treatment and suggested that it be tried for at least three months whenever an episode of nonbacterial prostatitis occurs.

However, critics of the allopurinol treatment contend that there is no clear evidence to support allopurinol's ability to relieve prostatitis. Also, some of the studies have found that the effects of allopurinol appear to wear off after about three months. Many men with prostatitis who've tried allopurinol have been disappointed.

Still, if you have a recurring case of nonbacterial prostatitis that refuses to respond to any other treatment, you may want to ask your doctor about trying allopurinol. Since allopurinol may affect PSA levels, ask your doctor about recording your base PSA levels before you begin treatment.

Tip-offs to rip-offs

Unfortunately, experimenting with alternative medicine can be like leaping into murky waters filled with hungry piranhas. To protect yourself from being eaten alive, watch out for these red flags of fraud.

▶ A claim that a product works by a "secret formula."

▶ Ads in the back pages of magazines, phone solicitations, editorial style newspaper ads, and 30-minute television commercials.

▶ A claim that a product is an amazing or miraculous breakthrough. Real medical breakthroughs are rare. Most alternative medical practices that work have been around for a while.

▶ Guarantees of a quick, painless cure.

Steer clear of any alternative medicine doctor who wants you to stop seeing your regular doctor. He should want to work along with your regular doctor. Also, ask any practitioner of alternative therapy if he is certified.

Before you begin a treatment, try to find people who've gone through it already. Most people will be honest about their experiences.

Be open-minded — but wary, too.

In summary

If you suspect your prostate is at the root of your troubles but aren't sure just what kind of prostate problem you have, take the test called *Identify your prostate problem* at the beginning of this chapter. Although prostate problems are characterized primarily by pain, this test can help you decide if your problems are mostly irritative or obstructive.

If most of your symptoms are irritative, you probably have an infection. If you have almost equal amounts of irritative and obstructive symptoms, you may have an inflamed prostate or BPH.

But before you lay all the blame on your poor old prostate, you'll want to make sure it's not urethritis that's causing your pain. Urethritis is an inflammation of the urethra, which may be caused by an infection, an irritation, or a minor injury.

Symptoms include a watery discharge from your penis, a penis that appears glued shut, a brownish or yellowish stain on the front of your underwear, an itchy feeling inside your penis, or a feeling of discomfort in your penis during urination. Since urethritis is typically caused by an infection, antibiotics usually clear up this problem quickly.

Once you rule out BPH and urethritis, prostate pain is generally lumped into four main categories: acute bacterial prostatitis, chronic bacterial prostatitis, nonbacterial prostatitis, and prostatodynia.

Acute bacterial prostatitis is the least common of the four. It's also the easiest to diagnose and treat effectively. Symptoms include fever, chills, blood in the urine, lower back pain, and extremely urgent or painful urination. Four to six weeks of antibiotics will normally eliminate the infection, as well as reduce the risk of the infection becoming chronic.

Chronic bacterial prostatitis may progress from a case of acute bacterial prostatitis that was never completely cured. This condition also appears to be linked with repeated urinary tract infections (UTIs). In fact, unless you've had a case of acute bacterial prostatitis or a urinary tract infection, it's unlikely you have chronic bacterial prostatitis. Symptoms include painful, urgent, or frequent urination, as well as pain in the lower back and a feeling of pressure or heaviness behind the scrotum.

It typically takes 10 to 12 weeks of full-strength antibiotics to knock out a case of chronic bacterial prostatitis. Because it's difficult for antibiotics to penetrate the prostate, many doctors also recommend a maintenance course of antibiotics for several more months to be sure the infection is completely eliminated.

Nonbacterial prostatitis is the most common kind of prostatitis, occurring about eight times more often than any other type. Unfortunately, it is also the least understood. While the term "nonbacterial prostatitis" suggests that bacteria aren't to blame for this particular problem, researchers are no longer sure this is the case. Recent studies have turned up some difficult-to-detect bacteria in these so-called cases of nonbacterial prostatitis. This form of prostatitis often responds well to antibiotics, which provides additional support for the theory that bacteria may be to blame for this hard-to-treat and painful prostate problem.

Symptoms include pain in the perineum and painful, frequent, or urgent urination. Symptoms may also come and go without warning.

Doctors often treat nonbacterial prostatitis with antibiotics and drugs that relax the muscles of the prostate gland. There are also a wide variety of home remedies that may be helpful for this problem.

Prostatodynia is similar to nonbacterial prostatitis except that men diagnosed with this problem show no signs of either infection or inflammation in their prostates. (Men with nonbacterial prostatitis show clear signs of inflammation, although the signs of infection are much harder to detect.)

Meaning "painful prostate," prostatodynia is characterized by lower back pain and pain in the pelvic and genital areas. Doctors suspect this apparent prostate problem may actually be caused by bladder, pelvic, or rectal muscles that are overly tense or generally out of whack.

Most of the self-help suggestions for nonbacterial prostatitis are also helpful for prostatodynia. If those don't give you any relief, ask your doctor about muscle relaxants or antibiotics. Although doctors aren't sure if this disorder is caused by bacteria, antibiotics have given some men relief.

Whatever type of prostate problem you think you may have, it's important to always see a doctor. Although knowing what kinds of disorders may be causing your problems is helpful when discussing your situation with your doctor, you need to let your doctor make the final diagnosis.

Untreated or misdiagnosed disorders can lead to worse problems, such as a urethral stricture or a chronic case of prostatitis, which can be very painful. The sooner you see a doctor, the better your chances for a cure and a complete recovery.

If my wife hadn't urged me to call the doctor,
I still wouldn't know I had benign prostate disease.
Johnny Unitas, winner of two NFL titles

4

Benign prostatic hyperplasia (BPH)

Difficulty getting urine stream to start; hesitancy

Weak urine stream

Feeling of incomplete emptying after urination

Frequent need to urinate

Having to get up one or more times during the night to urinate

Dribbling, incontinence

Insomnia

Interruptions in urine stream

There's BPH that's just bothersome, and then there's BPH that's bad like you never wanted it to be. If your BPH gets bad enough, neither your wife nor anyone else will need to urge you to call your doctor. You probably won't be able to get there fast enough.

Even if all your symptoms suggest BPH that is just a bother, see your doctor for a professional diagnosis. Not all bladder problems signal BPH. What may seem like symptoms of BPH are sometimes caused by other disorders, such as gonorrhea, bladder cancer or stones, diabetes, Parkinson's disease, multiple sclerosis, sexual problems, or even prostate cancer. Without a correct diagnosis, you won't be able to give your body the care it needs.

Although BPH can cause serious urinary and kidney problems by interfering with the flow of urine, this is not usually the case. The good news is having BPH does not make you more likely to get prostate cancer, although you can have both conditions.

Usually, an enlarged prostate is not a life-threatening problem. However, if it causes urine retention, it can lead to a bladder or kidney infection. Occasionally, the bladder muscles will fail completely from the constant effort of trying to push urine through a blocked passageway. Symptoms may come and go, depending on weather, stress levels, and other factors.

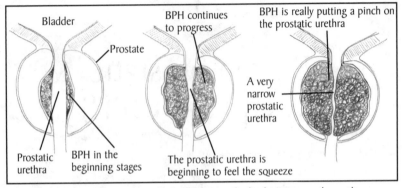

Figure 4.1 - BPH in progress. As cells continue to multiply, they squeeze the urethra more and more, usually making it much more difficult to urinate.

What is BPH?

Benign prostatic hyperplasia, also called BPH, is a non-cancerous condition that affects half the men over age 60 and 90 percent of men 85 years and older. Actually, most men are affected by BPH whether they notice any symptoms or not.

BPH begins when the number of prostate cells starts to increase. Eventually, if enough cells multiply, your prostate will enlarge. Problems occur because the enlarged prostate presses on the urethra (the tube that transports urine from the bladder to the penis and out of the body) and prevents your bladder from being emptied completely. This leads to annoying symptoms like dribbling, a slow stream, and having to urinate a lot more often than you used to.

The size of your prostate does not always determine how severe your symptoms are. Some men with really enlarged glands have little obstruction and few symptoms, while others whose glands are less enlarged have more blockage and worse problems.

You may be annoyed by your BPH, but you're not alone. In addition to the majority of men around you, both Benjamin

Franklin and Thomas Jefferson suffered from this condition. BPH may be a bother, but it isn't a barrier to continued success and enjoyment. Take the example of Franklin and Jefferson as your inspiration. Both lived productive lives until their early 80s in an era when you were lucky to live to be 60.

Spare yourself unnecessary surgery

When urine can't get through your urethra, it has no place to go but back up into your bladder. There it often stagnates and makes urinary tract and bladder infections more likely. You may also develop painful bladder stones or experience sexual difficulties.

Untreated BPH can even lead to kidney damage because of increased pressure on the kidneys or the spread of infection from the bladder to the kidneys. Sometimes, the urethra is squeezed so tightly by the prostate that it becomes impossible to urinate. This is called acute urinary retention, and it requires immediate medical attention.

Things that can trigger urinary retention include delaying urination, urinary tract infection, alcohol intake, antidepressants, decongestants, tranquilizers, cold temperatures, and being still for long periods of time.

If you have this problem, worry about what caused it later. Right now, see a doctor immediately! Normally, your doctor will relieve the retention by inserting a catheter (a slender, hollow tube) into your urethra and up to your bladder to drain it.

Be sure to tell your doctor if you've been taking any over-the-counter cold or allergy medicines. Such medicines contain a decongestant drug, known as a sympathomimetic, which causes problems in some men by preventing the bladder opening from relaxing and allowing urine to empty. Sometimes, simply switching to a different cold or allergy medicine can clear up your symptoms completely.

If you don't tell your doctor about all the medicines you're taking, both prescribed and over-the-counter, you run the risk of being railroaded into a surgery you don't need. Every year about one-third of men with urinary retention caused by over-the-counter medicines or constipation undergo prostatectomies for an enlarged prostate. All they really needed was a catheter to drain the bladder and to switch or stop using the medicines causing their problems.

Save yourself from the stress of an unnecessary surgery. Tell your doctor about all the drugs you're taking, whether they're prescribed or not.

Shrink your risk of BPH

Doctors aren't entirely sure what causes BPH. For centuries, they've known that BPH occurs mainly in older men and that it doesn't develop in men whose testes were removed before puberty. For this reason, some researchers believe that factors related to aging and the testes may spur the development of BPH.

Throughout their lives, men produce both testosterone, an important male hormone, and small amounts of estrogen, a female hormone. As men age, the amount of active testosterone in the blood decreases, leaving a higher proportion of estrogen. Studies suggest that BPH may occur because the higher amount of estrogen within the gland promotes cell growth and thus enlargement of the prostate.

Another theory focuses on dihydrotestosterone (DHT), a substance derived from testosterone in the prostate which may help control its growth. Some research has indicated that even with a drop in the blood's testosterone level, older men continue to produce and accumulate high levels of DHT in the prostate. This accumulation of DHT may encourage the growth of cells. Scientists have also noted that men who do not produce DHT do not develop BPH.

Other researchers suggest that BPH may develop as a result of "instructions" given to cells early in life. According to this theory, BPH occurs because cells in one section of the gland follow these instructions and "reawaken" later in life. These "reawakened" cells then deliver signals to other cells in the gland, instructing them to grow or making them more sensitive to hormones that influence growth.

There's not much you can do about growing older or how your hormones behave in your body. However, a recent study suggests you may have a little more control over another possible risk factor for BPH — how much you weigh.

According to a five-year study of more than 25,000 men, being 35 pounds or more overweight or gaining more than 7 inches in your waist increases your risk of BPH by 75 percent

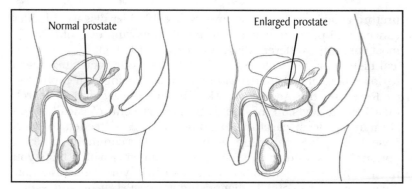

Figure 4.2 - Normal prostate vs. enlarged prostate.

after age 50. In fact, by age 75 to 80, about half the men with a waist size larger than 43 inches had moderate to severe urinary problems with some of them even requiring surgery. On the other hand, only about one-third of the men with a waist size of 35 inches or less had significant urinary difficulties.

Dr. Edward Giovannucci, author of the study, suggests that the extra stomach fat may press against the prostate gland, causing the problems with urination. Another possibility is that the extra fat raises estrogen levels while lowering testosterone levels. The extra estrogen promotes prostate growth.

How to get the right diagnosis

Before your doctor starts the physical exam, he'll want to hear about your medical history in detail, including any surgeries you've had. Specifically, he'll want to know if you've had problems with your urinary system and how healthy you are in general. If you keep a urination diary, take it with you. It can be a great help to your doctor in determining what's causing your problems. You may also find it handy to make a list of your symptoms before your visit. That way you won't be likely to forget any.

Generally, your doctor will be able to diagnose BPH based on your symptoms and a digital rectal exam. However, the urinary symptoms commonly seen in men with BPH are broad and can apply to various diseases. Urinary tract infection, narrowing of the urethra called urethral stricture disease, bladder disease, bladder cancer, and prostate cancer can mimic the symptoms of BPH. In most cases, the different diagnoses can be ruled out by your medical history or the basic exam. Sometimes, your doctor may need to do additional tests to determine what is causing your problems.

Recently, the Agency for Health Care Policy and Research (AHCPR), a division of the U.S. Department of Health and Human Services, carefully examined the tests needed to diagnose BPH. They came up with a list of recommended tests, optional tests, and unnecessary tests. Knowing which tests you need to have and which you don't can help you determine how effectively your doctor is diagnosing your BPH. If he suggests a test the AHCPR says you really don't need, ask him specifically why you need that test. If he can't give you a satisfactory answer, you may want to consider another doctor. For a complete description of these tests, see Chapter 14.

Recommended tests. Most doctors use these tests to diagnose BPH:

- Medical history

- Physical exam

- Digital rectal exam

- Urinalysis

- Measurement of serum creatinine

- Symptom assessment test (See the chart *Rate your BPH symptoms*)

Optional tests. Some doctors like to use these tests to verify their diagnoses and/or try to predict the results of treatment:

- Prostate specific antigen (PSA) test

- Uroflowmetry

- Pressure-flow studies

- Residual urine measurement

- Urethrocystoscopy (appropriate if invasive treatments are planned)

Unnecessary tests:

- Ultrasonography or urogram

- Cystometry

- Urethrocystoscopy (not recommended as a way to determine need for treatment)

PSA testing: optional or indispensable?

When the AHCPR published its guidelines for treating BPH, which includes the list of recommended, optional, and unnecessary tests, some doctors definitely disagreed with their recommendations.

The part that some doctors protested was the AHCPR's decision to list the PSA test as optional for diagnosing BPH.

The doctors who disagreed say the PSA test is essential to rule out prostate cancer before making a diagnosis of BPH. Among those who objected are Dr. William Catalona, department chief of urology at Washington University School of Medicine in St. Louis, Mo., and Dr. Abraham Crockett, former president of the American Urological Association.

So why did the AHCPR decide to call the PSA test optional?

According to Dr. John McConnell, head of the 13-member panel who created the guidelines, the panel classified the test as optional because BPH also elevates PSA levels, which theoretically could lead to a false-positive diagnosis of cancer, resulting in more unnecessary tests.

The panel also points out that detecting prostate cancer in older men who have other health problems may be more harmful than helpful. For those men, the rigors and side effects of treatment may not extend their life spans enough to make compromising the quality of their remaining years worth it. In fact, studies suggest that early diagnosis of prostate cancer may not improve the eventual outcome or prolong life in many men. Other, more recent studies suggest the PSA test does benefit some men.

However, when it's your life that's on the line, it's easy to see those studies in an entirely different light. That's why whether or not you have the PSA test should be a personal decision between you and your doctor.

Rate your BPH symptoms

If you want to know how your BPH symptoms measure up, take this test. Based on the International Prostate Screening Score (IPSS), it will help you determine if your symptoms are

	Points	0
Question		Not at all
Over the past month, how often have you had a sensation of not emptying your bladder completely after you finished urinating?		
Over the past month, how often have you had to urinate again less than two hours after you finished urinating?		
Over the past month, how often have you found you stopped and started again several times when you urinated?		
Over the past month, how often have you found it difficult to postpone urination?		
Over the past month, how often have you had a weak urinary stream?		
Over the past month, how often have you had to push or strain to begin urination?		
		None
Over the past month, how many times did you most typically get up to urinate from the time you went to bed at night until the time you got up in the morning?		

Add up each answer you circled to get your total score. If your score is 0 to 7, your symptoms are mild. If your score is 8 to 19,

mild, moderate, or severe. Many doctors also use this test to help them determine which treatment options would give you the most relief. They may also use it later to evaluate how well your chosen treatment is working for you.

1	2	3	4	5
Less than 1 in 5	Less than half the time	About half the time	More than half the time	Almost always
1 time	2 times	3 times	4 times	5 or more times

you have moderate BPH. If your score is 20 to 35, you're suffering from very severe symptoms.

Reprinted with permission from International Consultation of Urologic Diseases.

Treatment options:

Mild (0 to 7) — Although you will want to have your doctor recheck the progress of your BPH once a year, your only reasonable option is watchful waiting, (simply monitoring your symptoms while postponing treatment as long as possible). For mild symptoms, the risks of other treatments outweigh any possible benefits.

Moderate (8 to 19) — Even if your symptoms are moderate, there's no need to automatically assume the worst. You have a wide variety of treatment options open to you, including watchful waiting, 5-alpha-reductase inhibitors, alpha adrenergic antagonists, microwave therapy, laser prostatectomy, stents, TUIP, and TURP. In addition, a review of five studies found that among men with moderate BPH who chose watchful waiting and were followed for five years, about 40 percent improved and 45 percent stayed the same. Only 15 percent got worse.

Severe (20 to 35) — Treatment options include 5-alpha-reductase inhibitors, alpha adrenergic antagonists, microwave therapy, laser prostatectomy, stents, TUIP, TURP, and open prostatectomy.

Bettin' on BPH

If you've charted the location of every men's room from Maine to New Mexico and everywhere in between, chances are you're suffering from BPH, a common condition affecting many men over the age of 50. "Benign" means the condition is not cancerous. "Hyperplasia" means there are more cells than normal.

Tracking down the right treatment for you

The AHCPR created this flow chart to help you and your doctor decide where you want to go from here with your BPH treatment.

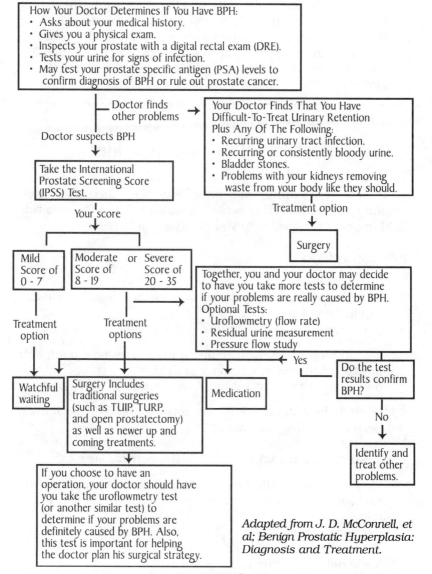

Figure 4.3 - AHCPR flow chart

It's a family thing

One family member diagnosed with BPH increases the risk that other male members of that family will develop the disorder as well. If your family member was diagnosed before age 60, this appears to slightly increase the risk that other family members will develop BPH. The risk appears the greatest in men who've had both a father and a brother with BPH, instead of just a father.

How does BPH affect your life?

In addition to rating their symptoms, some men also find it helpful to rate how BPH affects their quality of life. The following BPH Impact Index will help you determine just that.

BPH Impact Index

1. Over the past month, how much physical discomfort did any urinary problems cause you? _____
   0 = none   1 = only a little   2 = some   3 = a lot

2. Over the past month, how much did you worry about your health because of any urinary problems? _____
   0 = none   1 = only a little   2 = some   3 = a lot

3. Overall, how bothersome has any trouble with urination been during the past month? _____
   0 = not at all bothersome   2 = bothers me some
   1 = bothers me a little   3 = bothers me a lot

4. Over the past month, how much of the time has any urinary problem kept you from doing the kinds of things you would usually do? _____
   0 = none of the time   3 = most of the time
   1 = a little of the time   4 = all the time
   2 = some of the time

Add up the numbers of each response you circled to get your score.

BPH Impact Index Score = _____

The higher your score, the more negatively BPH impacts your life.

BPH treatments: Know your options

To decide which, if any, BPH treatment is best for you, work with your doctor to determine how bothered you are by your symptoms. Men with the same symptoms often feel quite differently about how much those symptoms bother them. That's why it's so important that you decide for yourself which treatment option you prefer without leaving the decision to your doctor. Your doctor will probably base his decision on an average of how other men have felt and responded to treatment. This could be very different from how you feel and respond.

You also need to decide how you feel about the possible risks and benefits of each treatment option. Ask your doctor these questions about each treatment:

- What are my chances of getting better?

- How much better will I get?

- What are the chances that the treatment will cause problems?

- How long will the treatment work?

Take an active role in choosing your treatment plan. According to a five-year study supported by the AHCPR, that's the best way to lower your chances of having prostate surgery you could potentially avoid.

Many doctors have access to video and computer programs that present the risks and benefits of different types of treatment in an easy-to-understand format. The programs feature men who've experienced good as well as bad outcomes after having prostate treatment. Some men find using the computer/video programs gives them a clearer idea of which option they'd like to choose.

Before choosing a treatment, ask yourself these important questions:

- If my BPH is not likely to cause me serious harm, do I want any treatment other than watchful waiting?

- If I do want treatment, which is the best for me based on the benefits and risks of each?

Discuss whatever you decide with your doctor. Ask any questions you have. Take this book with you for handy guidance. Together, you and your doctor can choose the best treatment for you.

Watchful waiting

Many men with less severe symptoms opt for "watchful waiting," which is merely monitoring symptoms carefully while postponing treatment as long as possible. If your symptoms are fairly mild and your IPSS score was seven or less, watchful waiting is probably a good option for you. Of course, you'll want to be rechecked annually to see how your symptoms are doing.

Generally, this is not dangerous. It rarely leads to any serious problems, such as urinary retention or renal failure, as some doctors originally thought. Even better news is that symptoms clear up on their own in one-third of men with mild cases of BPH.

In fact, watchful waiting is probably the best option for men who aren't very bothered by their urinary symptoms or who wish to put off surgery. Keep in mind that watchful waiting doesn't just mean sitting back and twiddling your thumbs. There are some things you can do in the meantime to make yourself much more comfortable.

- ▶ Avoid tranquilizers and over-the-counter cold and sinus remedies that contain decongestants. They can make urination symptoms worse.

- ▶ Limit caffeine and alcohol and other prostate irritants, especially in late afternoon and near bedtime.

- ▶ Take time to urinate, rather than rushing.

- ▶ If you use anticholinergics or diuretics, ask your doctor about switching to a different drug.

In addition to these tips, always have a yearly exam to check the progress of your BPH symptoms just to make sure your kidneys and bladder are still in good shape.

Managing BPH with medicine

The fact that your prostate is made up of two different kinds of tissue, glandular and smooth muscle, affects how drugs work to relieve your BPH.

The glandular part of your prostate produces fluid that makes up some of your semen. Your prostate's smooth muscle squeezes this fluid out into the urethra where it mixes with sperm and other stuff that make up semen.

Just as the two different types of tissue have different jobs to do, they have different ways of affecting your prostate once it begins to enlarge. Glandular tissue actually grows to the point where it blocks your urethra. Then, when the smooth muscle tissue contracts, it squeezes your urethra and stops urination.

The two major types of drugs used to treat BPH are alpha blockers and finasteride (Proscar). Finasteride focuses on glandular tissue problems, slowing tissue growth and sometimes even shrinking your prostate to unblock your urethra.

The alpha blockers take a different approach. They actually relax the smooth muscles that are squeezing your urethra tighter and tighter, making it harder and harder for urine to get through. Once your smooth muscles get the signal to relax, urine has a much easier time going through your urethra.

Alpha blocker drug treatment

Originally intended to treat high blood pressure, researchers have also found that alpha blockers can relieve BPH symptoms by relaxing the tightened muscles of the enlarged prostate. These drugs seem to be most beneficial for men with mild to moderate symptoms. Most men notice improvement within four to six weeks.

One study found that alpha blockers relieve symptoms in 70 percent of men taking it, compared to only 40 percent of men taking a placebo (a fake pill). Another study found that it improved symptoms in two out of three men. However, there is no evidence that alpha blockers reduce the rate of BPH complications or the need for future surgery.

Alpha blockers include doxazosin (Cardura), prazosin (Minipress), terazosin (Hytrin), and tamsulosin (Flomax).

You take alpha blockers by mouth, usually once or twice a day. During your first three or four weeks on these drugs, you'll probably need to see your doctor regularly so he can monitor your progress. Normally, he increases your dose gradually to lessen side effects. If you take other drugs for high blood pressure, your dose of alpha blockers may need to be adjusted.

In fact, if you need drugs for high blood pressure, your doctor may be able to use terazosin to treat both your BPH and your high blood pressure at the same time. Studies have found that terazosin effectively treats BPH while lowering systolic blood pressure (the top number in a blood pressure reading) by 4 to 18 points.

Side effects may include headaches, dizziness, tiredness, and low blood pressure. In people with heart disease, alpha blockers may cause chest pains. Rarely, alpha blockers can cause retrograde ejaculation (where semen backs up into the bladder instead of being forced out through the penis) by relaxing the bladder neck a little too much. Because alpha blocker treatment for BPH is new, doctors don't know its long-term risks and benefits.

Finasteride drug treatment

Finasteride relieves BPH symptoms by actually shrinking the prostate. This drug works by blocking the conversion of testosterone to dihydrotestosterone, which tends to promote prostate enlargement.

Finasteride falls into the drug category of androgen suppressants or anti-androgens. Anti-androgens work to relieve BPH by blocking testosterone from binding with receptors in the prostate, which encourages the prostate to grow. (Testosterone is a type of androgen, which is just a general term for any male hormone. Blocking testosterone means blocking androgen, which is how researchers came up with the term anti-androgen treatment.)

If dihydrotestosterone levels decrease, the prostate shrinks. After about 12 months on this drug, 30 percent of men show some improvement in symptoms.

Although finasteride can shrink the prostate 25 to 30 percent, it may take four months to a year before you notice any benefit. Studies suggest that this drug is only effective in men whose prostates are larger than 40 centimeters (cm). Unlike alpha blockers, there is now evidence that finasteride reduces the rate of BPH complications and the need for future surgery.

In a recent study of 2,760 men, researchers found that men who took 5 mg of finasteride a day for four years had a 55 percent reduced risk of surgery and a 57 percent reduced risk of acute urinary retention compared with men who took a placebo.

Although these figures look good, you need to keep a couple of points in mind before you rush off to your doctor to request finasteride. Finasteride seems to be most effective in men who have large prostates with moderate to severe BPH and low urinary flow rates.

If you don't fit that profile exactly, you may want to ponder on Proscar for a bit (the brand name for finasteride). Even among men with that profile, urinary symptoms tend to worsen slowly if at all. Chances are good you may not need the preventive care Proscar can provide. This means you could waste approximately $700 per year on a drug that really doesn't offer you that many benefits. It's also not known how much finasteride will improve your quality of life.

You take finasteride by mouth once a day, and you'll need to see your doctor regularly while you're taking this drug.

Side effects may include less interest in sex, as well as erection and ejaculation problems. Be sure that any woman in your life also uses caution around this drug, especially if she is pregnant or possibly pregnant. Studies show that pregnant women, or women planning to become pregnant, who are exposed to crushed or broken finasteride tablets (or the semen of a man taking finasteride) risk exposing their male fetuses and causing birth defects.

In addition, finasteride lowers the blood levels of PSA. Doctors often measure your PSA levels to determine your risk of prostate cancer. Your doctor will need to take your use of this drug into account when evaluating your PSA test results. Generally, if you've been taking finasteride for six months or more, your doctor can multiply your PSA reading by two to get an accurate estimate of your true PSA level.

Treat your BPH and beat baldness, too

By age 80 almost all men are facing a double whammy — both BPH and baldness. Many men must face these unpleasant facts of life as early as age 50 and some as soon as age 30. But wait, there is good news. You may be able to beat these two bad "B's" with one little pill.

Researchers noticed that some of the men taking finasteride (Proscar) for an enlarged prostate also started growing new hair on their heads. Most of the new hair growth occurred on top of the head at the front of the scalp.

Researchers were excited to find that finasteride stimulates actual new hair growth instead of the fuzz that some hair regrowth products produce. Even if you fail to grow new hair while you're taking finasteride, researchers think it will prevent any future hair loss.

However, don't expect to grow back all the hair you've lost. Although finasteride does increase the number of scalp hairs, which will help fill in thin or balding spots, it won't replace all the scalp hairs you've shed over the years. Also, you have to keep taking finasteride for these benefits to last. They wear off about a year after you stop taking the drug. The bad news is that if you were totally bald to begin with, you shouldn't pin all your hopes on finasteride. It won't help a whit.

Basically, finasteride works the same way to stop male-pattern baldness as it does to shrink an enlarged prostate. It interferes with the body's conversion of testosterone to dihydrotestosterone. Researchers believe it is this conversion of testosterone that contributes to both prostate enlargement and male-pattern baldness.

Men who don't have enlarged prostates but still want to see if this new drug can stop their hair loss can try it out in the form of a prescription for Propecia, the brand name for the dosage of finasteride used to treat hair loss. If you already take finasteride for an enlarged prostate, just consider the hair growth an added plus.

Which drug does the best job?

At this time, the two most preferred drugs for treating BPH are alpha blockers and finasteride. Is one better than the other?

Well, researchers have been busy trying to determine just that. According to their most recent findings comparing the two drugs, terazosin (an alpha blocker) is tops.

In a one-year, double-blind, placebo-controlled study (the most reliable type of study) of 1,229 men with BPH, researchers compared terazosin, finasteride, and a combination of the two drugs.

According to the study's results, terazosin takes first place in relieving symptoms of BPH. Finasteride wasn't any better than a placebo. The combination of terazosin and finasteride rated slightly better, but the researchers say the difference wasn't significant.

Critics of the study maintain that finasteride really wasn't given a fair shake. Finasteride's developers say the drug works best in men with prostates larger than 40 mm. The men in this study had prostates averaging from 37.2 to 38.4 mm.

A new study — the largest, longest, and most expensive study ever conducted on BPH — also found that finasteride decreases the risk of urinary retention as well as the need for surgery.

Although terazosin may work better for the majority of men, the drug that does you the most good may ultimately depend on the size of your prostate. If one of these two drugs doesn't work for you, consider trying the other or a combination of the two.

Get the facts on traditional treatments

The chart on the following page gives you a quick overview of the pros and cons of the most traditional BPH treatments, except for surgery.

For a complete discussion of surgery options for BPH, as well as a complete description of new and upcoming treatments, see Chapter 5.

Pros and cons of traditional BPH treatments

Treatment	Chances of symptom improvement	Risk of dying within 3 months of treatment
Watchful waiting	Unknown	—
Alpha blockers	51%	—
Finasteride	31%	—

* Mainly from visits to doctor's office.
— No data available.
1. Calculated from Medicare data (1988-89) and drug and device cost estimates.

Sexual survival guide

Does BPH slam the brakes on sex?

Not at all, according to several recent studies.

Of course, as some men get older they do experience sexual problems and many find it convenient to blame BPH.

However, these studies say that BPH should not bear the brunt of the blame. Researchers found that the apparent increase in sexual problems in men who have BPH actually parallels the overall increase in impotence in the general population. Basically, that means as men get older they tend to develop impotence, probably as a result of other health problems, but not necessarily BPH.

On the other hand, even though BPH itself doesn't generally cause a problem, some of the treatments used for BPH can increase your risk of impotence or other sexual problems. If remaining potent is a priority in your life, keep it in mind when choosing a treatment.

Of the different drugs used to treat BPH, finasteride is the one most likely to cause sexual difficulties. Common complaints include impotence, loss of desire, and a decreased amount of ejaculate.

Aside from complications caused by finasteride, the most common sexual problem of BPH treatment is retrograde ejaculation.

Risk of complications	Total incontinence	Hospital stay	Loss of work time	Cost (1,2)
1 - 5% from BPH progression	None	0	1 day*	$1,162.00
3 - 43%	None	0	3.5 days*	$1,395.00
14 - 19%	None	0	1.5 days*	$1,326.00

2. Estimates for watchful waiting, finasteride, and alpha blockers are probably higher than those actually seen because not all men choose surgery if these treatments fail.

This doesn't affect your ability to have sex, although you may experience a slightly different sensation.

However, retrograde ejaculation does render most men infertile, so this can be a problem for men who hope to father children. But for most men with BPH, it's hardly more than a nuisance.

The surgeries most likely to cause retrograde ejaculation include prostatectomy and transurethral resection of the prostate (TURP), also known as transurethral prostatectomy. Transurethral incision of the prostate (TUIP) poses a much lower risk of this problem. Even if you do become infertile after BPH treatment, you may still be able to father children with a little help from your doctor. Many times, it is possible to retrieve sperm from your bladder and use them to artificially inseminate your mate.

Of much greater importance to most men is the risk of impotence. To find out which treatments pose the greatest and least risks, see the following chart.

Keep in mind these numbers represent the *average* risk and your risk may be higher or lower depending on your health, age, and other factors. Talk over your options with your doctor carefully before making a choice.

BPH treatments and sex: Weighing the risks

Treatment	Retrograde ejaculation	Impotence
Alpha blockers	6.2%	Probably no added risk
Finasteride	0%	2.5 to 5.3%
TUIP	24.9%	11.7%
TURP	73.4%	13.6%
Prostatectomy	77.2% (supraretro)	4.7 to 39.2%
Retropubic prostatectomy*	—	16.2%
Suprapubic prostatectomy*	—	17.7%

* All types of the traditional prostatectomy. Retropubic and suprapubic simply refer to the different areas of your body surgeons may go through in order to reach your prostate.
– No data available.

Everything you need to know about natural remedies

In Europe, at least 30 compounds containing active ingredients from plants are used to treat BPH. In 70 percent of studies, plants have been found to be more effective than a placebo. In fact, some studies suggest plant remedies may help up to 80 percent of the men using them. The major advantage of plant remedies over manufactured drugs is the much lower risk of serious side effects.

Here are some of the more common remedies used to treat BPH. Their botanical names are listed in parentheses after the common names. If you choose to use any of these remedies, be sure you let your doctor know. He will still need to regularly check how your BPH is doing.

Also, if you buy any of these products, look for ones labeled "standardized." That means the manufacturer has tried to get a consistent amount of the healing herb in each pill. You may find several of these plants sold in combination products. This is because manufacturers hope that by combining the different plants, they may be able to provide a more potent remedy.

Saw palmetto (*Serenoa repens*). A small palm tree that grows in the southeastern United States could help relieve your BPH. Several studies found that a concentrated extract of saw palmetto berries is at least as effective as finasteride in treating BPH. Several other small studies suggest saw palmetto may be as effective as alpha blockers, too.

One study found that men with BPH who took saw palmetto for three months had more than twice the urine flow of men who took finasteride for a year. Other studies have reported that saw palmetto may help up to 80 percent of the men using this remedy. However, critics of the saw palmetto studies suggest the study designs favor saw palmetto.

About 5 percent of the people taking saw palmetto report side effects, most commonly gastrointestinal symptoms like nausea, constipation, and diarrhea. About 5 percent of men taking finasteride also report side effects. However, the side effects of finasteride include impotence, incontinence, and decreased sexual drive. Most men would probably rather deal with diarrhea.

Supporters of saw palmetto say it works by interfering with the production of dihydrotestosterone, a hormone that promotes prostate growth. In addition to being safe and about as effective, saw palmetto's cost is only one-third that of the leading prescription drug for BPH. Both French and German health authorities have already approved saw palmetto to treat enlarged prostates.

In order to be effective, saw palmetto must contain the fat-soluble parts of the plant. This means that drinking saw palmetto in the form of a tea won't help you because it doesn't contain enough active ingredients from the berry to be useful.

If you want to try saw palmetto, check out your local health food store or herb shop and choose a supplement of lipophilic (fat-soluble) extract that contains fatty acids. Make sure any brand you choose contains 85 to 95 percent fatty acids. Experts recommend taking 160 milligrams (mg) twice daily or 320 mg once a day. It may take four to six weeks before you notice any improvement. Use it as long as it gives you relief.

There is some concern that saw palmetto may decrease PSA levels. If this is indeed the case, it could interfere with the detection of cancer. Although the most recent research suggests that saw palmetto really has no effect on PSA levels, just to be on the safe side you may want to get a baseline measurement of your PSA level before you start taking saw palmetto.

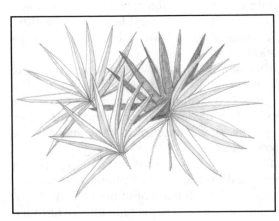

Figure 4.4 - Saw palmetto

The story of saw palmetto

Although researchers have only recently begun to rally support for saw palmetto's ability to relieve BPH, it's been a staple of the human diet for centuries.

However, harvesting this reddish-brown, slightly wrinkled berry is only for the hardy. Harvesters have to brave the razor sharp teeth of the saw palmetto plant and trek through areas that alligators and eastern diamond-back rattlers like to haunt.

Despite the harvesting hazards, the early inhabitants of South Florida centered their diet around the nutritious little berry. (The Seminole Indians preferred it more for its supposed powers as an aphrodisiac.)

Saw palmetto didn't have quite the same appeal for early Europeans. A group of Quakers shipwrecked on the southern coast of Florida in the late 1700s compared the sweet-bitter taste of the saw palmetto berry to "rotten cheese steeped in tobacco juice." Eventually, though, the Quakers learned to tolerate the taste in order to save themselves from starvation.

Dr. J.B. Read of Savannah, Ga., was the first to sing the praises of saw palmetto in a medical publication, the *American Journal of Pharmacy*. In 1879, he wrote that saw palmetto "induces sleep, relieves the most troublesome coughs ... improves digestion, and increases fat, flesh, and strength."

But it wasn't until 1892 that anyone noted the berry's beneficial effects on the reproductive organs. A doctor whose letter appeared in the July 1892 edition of *The New Idea* wrote, "It [saw palmetto] also exerts a great influence over the organs of reproduction — mammaries, ovarium, prostate, testes, etc. ..."

By the late 1920s, doctors began to recognize saw palmetto's direct influence on the bladder, prostate, and urethra. The 1926 edition of the United States Dispensatory noted, "It has been especially recommended in cases of enlarged prostate. ..."

Unfortunately, as researchers learned how to make more potent drugs synthetically, saw palmetto fell out of favor in the United States as a treatment for BPH.

However, a long history of use in European countries, as well as several studies that provide convincing support for saw palmetto's effectiveness, have revived an interest in the prickly plant. This time it looks like saw palmetto may be here to stay.

Stinging nettle (*Urtica dioica*). The root of the stinging nettle plant may be able to put the sting to urinary difficulties commonly caused by BPH. In addition, its leaves may also increase urinary flow.

The usual way to consume nettle leaves is in a tea made with three to four teaspoonfuls of nettle. Some herbal experts recommend drinking a cup of this tea three to four times daily or taking a supplement — 120 mg twice daily.

You may also want to try taking a combination of saw palmetto and nettle root. One study of 2,080 men found that the combo of 160 mg of saw palmetto and 120 mg of stinging nettle root extract taken twice a day improved urinary flow by 26 percent, reduced residual urine (urine left in the bladder after you urinate) by 45 percent, reduced pain during urination by 63 percent, reduced dribbling after urination by 54 percent, and cut nighttime trips to the bathroom by half.

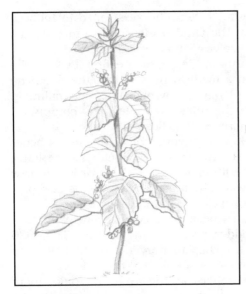

Figure 4.5 - Stinging nettle

African plum (*Pygeum africanum*). The bark of the *pygeum africanum* tree, which grows in tropical Africa, is used to make an extract for the treatment of BPH and prostatitis. Besides relieving your BPH symptoms, it may improve sexual performance in some men with prostate disorders.

The recommended amount is 50 to 100 mg of a *pygeum* supplement twice daily. Because some manufacturers believe saw palmetto and African plum work well together, you'll probably find *pygeum* sold in combination products as well.

You may also find *pygeum* and needle root sold together. At least one study has found that needle root and *pygeum* work better in combination than either one does separately.

Rye grass pollen (*Secale cereale*). Rye grass pollen comes from the pollen of a few specially classified plants growing in southern Sweden. Well-designed scientific studies have revealed that it significantly reduces nighttime urination as well as daytime trips to the bathroom.

Many of the rye grass pollen studies have been done using a product called Cernilton. If you'd prefer that brand over others, you can buy Cernilton from Cernitin America by calling (800) 831-9505.

South African star grass (*Hypoxis rooperi*). Star grass is found in South Africa, South America, Australia, and Asia. The active principle of the plant, sitosterol, comes from its root.

Although this is probably the most popular product used to treat BPH in Germany, studies on its effectiveness are conflicting. A very reliable controlled study reported significant measurable improvement in the rate of urine flow (as opposed to improvement simply reported but not measured).

Another equally reliable study found no difference between *Hypoxis rooperi* and a placebo. In an uncontrolled study (one of the least reliable study methods), researchers noted that 39 percent of the men taking *Hypoxis rooperi* became symptom-free and 53 percent improved.

Pumpkin seeds (*Cucurbita pepo*). Researchers have found that the seeds of this plant can slightly improve the urine flow in men with BPH. A handful of pumpkin seeds a day is a popular remedy for an enlarged prostate in Bulgaria, Turkey, and the Ukraine.

One study of a combination of saw palmetto and pumpkin seed extracts was shown to improve urine flow as well as significantly reduce the number of times men needed to urinate during the day. It also reduced nighttime urination as well as pain during urination.

Amino acids. At least one study has reported a beneficial effect of a combination of the amino acids glycine, alanine, and glutamic acid in relieving the symptoms of BPH. In a placebo-controlled study of 40 men, researchers found that the glycine, alanine, glutamic acid capsules reduced prostate size and relieved symptoms of BPH including nighttime urination, delayed urination, frequent urination, and urgency.

During the study, the men took three capsules three times daily after meals for two weeks. After that, they took one capsule three times daily. Each capsule contained 6-1/4 grains of a mixture of glycine, alanine, and glutamic acid. No one experienced any adverse reactions to the amino acids.

Foods, vitamins, and minerals that offer relief

Soy foods. Researchers at the University of Wales College of Medicine in Great Britain found that soy isoflavones (hormone-like substances found in soy products) block testosterone conversion to dihydrotestosterone.

Soy seems to stop, or at least slow down, the process of prostate enlargement, which is what causes all your annoying urinary symptoms. Good soy sources include soybeans, soy milk, textured vegetable protein, and tofu.

Lignans. These hormone-like substances that come from plants appear to have a similar effect. Good sources of lignans include berries, whole grains, and licorice, but flaxseed is the best source of all.

For the most benefit, you need to make both soy products and lignans a lifelong part of your diet. In addition, eat a low-fat diet. Researchers are pretty sure a low-fat diet can cut your risk of prostate cancer, and some evidence suggests a low-fat diet may help you avoid BPH. Dietary fat appears to increase hormone production, which, in turn, may stimulate prostate growth. Researchers speculate that eating a low-fat diet would protect your prostate from these extra hormones.

Vitamin B6. Also known as pyridoxine, this vitamin enhances your body's absorption of zinc. Make sure you're getting at least 2 mg of B6 a day.

Selenium. Lab studies suggest selenium may inhibit the growth of prostate cells. The recommended dose is 100 micrograms (mcg) a day.

Zinc. Studies suggest zinc may help reduce the size of the prostate as well as relieve the symptoms of BPH. The recommended dose is 30 mg of zinc picolinate daily.

Mind over bladder

Healers have known for centuries that just having faith in a treatment is almost as important as the treatment itself. In fact, before antibiotics became available, doctors most commonly prescribed "little pink pills." Doctors found the pink pills worked better than others — presumably because their patients believed the pink pills packed the most powerful punch.

When it comes to controlling an unruly bladder, you have several options, but it may be your own mind that makes the most difference. Recent studies suggest the power of your mind appears to be especially effective for relieving the symptoms of BPH.

In a BPH study of over 600 men, 303 of those men received a placebo and 310 received the drug finasteride. Those who received the actual drug experienced fewer symptoms, as well as improved urine flow.

Amazingly enough, the placebo group also experienced faster urine flow and significant relief from their other symptoms. For the entire two years of the study, men with mild to moderate BPH symptoms continued to experience relief while taking the placebos. Interestingly enough, they also developed side effects, such as impotence and lack of interest in sex, they thought would be associated with the drugs.

How did this miraculous mind control work? Researchers speculate that the men's belief in the pills' ability to provide relief may have reduced nervous reactions that trigger smooth muscle contractions of the bladder, prostate, and urethra. The relaxed smooth muscles allowed urine to flow more easily.

You don't need medicine, fake or not, to fool your prostate into behaving better. Simply create an image in your mind of your prostate allowing your urine to flow easily. Practice recalling this image until it becomes routine. You may also gain more benefit from this technique, called visualization, if you take a class or read a book on the subject. Two good possibilities are *Creative Visualization* by Shakti Gawain and *Visualization for Change* by Patrick Fanning.

Whatever treatment you choose to use, believe it will work for you. You'll have a significantly greater shot at success.

In summary

Benign prostatic hyperplasia (BPH) is a common condition that affects half the men over age 60 and 90 percent of men 85 years and older. "Benign" means the condition is not cancerous.

"Hyperplasia" means there are more cells than normal. Both aging and hormones play a role in the development of BPH.

The process of BPH begins when the number of prostate cells starts to increase. Eventually, if enough cells multiply, your prostate will enlarge. Problems occur because the enlarged prostate presses on the urethra.

The enlarged prostate prevents your bladder from being emptied completely and leads to annoying symptoms like dribbling, a slow urine stream, and having to urinate a lot more often than you used to. However, these symptoms don't always signal BPH. That's why it's important to see your doctor for a diagnosis.

Untreated BPH can lead to kidney damage because of increased pressure on the kidneys and the spread of infection from the bladder to the kidneys. Sometimes, the urethra is squeezed so tightly by the prostate it becomes impossible to urinate. This is called acute urinary retention, and it requires immediate medical attention.

To diagnose BPH, most doctors rely on your medical history, a physical exam, a digital rectal exam, urinalysis, measurement of your serum creatinine (this test determines how well your kidneys are functioning), and your score on a written test of how much your symptoms bother you.

Generally, your choice of treatment will depend on how much discomfort you have. Options include watchful waiting, natural remedies, drug treatment, and surgery. Surgery is discussed in more detail in Chapters 5 and 6.

To decide which treatment is best for you, carefully weigh the pros and cons of each option discussed in this chapter. Unless symptoms are really severe, most men prefer to start with watchful waiting and natural therapies. Most men wait to try treatments that are likely to have the most severe side effects, such as drugs and surgery, until their symptoms worsen significantly or interfere with their overall health.

I got the bill for my surgery. Now I know what those doctors were wearing masks for.
James H. Boran, Professor of political science
and political humorist

5

BPH: The surgery solution

While it's true that surgery offers you the best chance at improving your urinary symptoms, it can also have the most severe side effects, including failure to improve symptoms or causing them to worsen. Impotence, incontinence, retrograde ejaculation (where semen backs up into the bladder instead of being forced out through the penis), and even death are possible complications.

For those reasons, most men prefer to save surgery as their last option. Even then, many men decide they can live with a little discomfort and inconvenience from BPH (benign prostatic hyperplasia) rather than accept the risks of surgery. As a general rule, men bothered by severe symptoms of BPH benefit most from surgery.

But don't choose surgery just because your doctor says your symptoms will get worse and your surgical risk will increase with age. The truth is that BPH symptoms progress slowly and even improve spontaneously in some cases. Since there is great variation among men with BPH, only you can determine how much your symptoms bother you.

However, some men simply don't have a choice. If you have a stubborn case of urinary retention (incomplete emptying of the bladder) that won't respond to catheter treatment, recurring urinary tract infections, urine that is frequently bloody, bladder stones, or kidney problems caused by BPH, most doctors will strongly recommend surgery as being in the best interest of your health.

Do you have a choice in the type of surgery you have? Experts suggest that the choice of surgery should be left up to the surgeon,

---

Surgery stats

In the United States alone, over 350,000 men have surgery each year to treat BPH. Transurethral prostatectomy (TURP) makes up the majority of these operations. Among people with Medicare, TURP is the second most commonly performed surgery, following closely behind cataract surgery. Costs for these surgeries range between $2 billion and $3 billion per year.

---

who will base his decision on the size and shape of your prostate gland. If he asks your preference and you have one, by all means feel free to express it, but don't be offended if you aren't consulted.

Types of surgery for BPH

Transurethral prostatectomy (TURP). This is the most common type of prostatectomy. More than 90 percent of prostates are removed by this method. Among surgeons, it is considered the "gold standard" of BPH surgical treatment, the one to which all the others are compared. Many doctors still insist that the worst prostate problems show the most improvement with TURP.

TURP can sometimes be done on an outpatient basis, although it usually requires a short hospital stay. If you can convince your doctor you're a good candidate for outpatient surgery, you'll probably save around $2,000.

To perform TURP, the surgeon passes a long, thin instrument called a resectoscope up through your urethra and into your bladder. The resectoscope contains a light, valves for controlling water to wash away excess tissue, and an electrical loop that cuts tissue and seals blood vessels.

During the 90-minute operation, the surgeon uses the resectoscope's wire loop to remove the excess tissue one piece at a time. The pieces of tissue are carried by the fluid into the bladder and then flushed out at the end of the operation. You will have to wear a catheter for 12 to 36 hours after surgery.

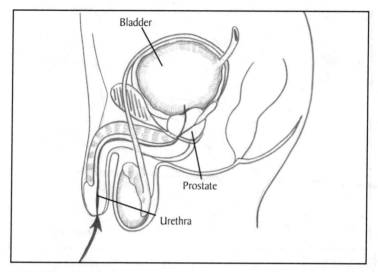

Figure 5.1 - The transurethral approach to the prostate. This is the route, up into the penis and through the urethra to the prostate, the surgeon takes when he performs a TURP or a TUIP.

Men usually recover quickly after a TURP, and it is generally very effective in relieving symptoms. However, some men experience side effects, such as narrowing of the urethra, urinary infection, bleeding, or retrograde ejaculation. About 5 to 10 percent experience impotence, and 2 to 4 percent have incontinence following surgery.

Other possible problems include infection and bleeding. Normally, antibiotics are prescribed to prevent an infection. In rare cases, a blood transfusion is required. See Chapter 6 for ways to reduce your risk of infection from a blood transfusion.

A few men undergoing TURP develop TURP syndrome. This rare complication occurs when the body absorbs too much of the water used to wash away excess prostate tissue. Symptoms include confusion, nausea, vomiting, high blood pressure, slow heart rate, and vision problems. This problem is only temporary and is treated using diuretics (water pills) or a saline solution to remove the extra fluid from the body and restore mineral balance.

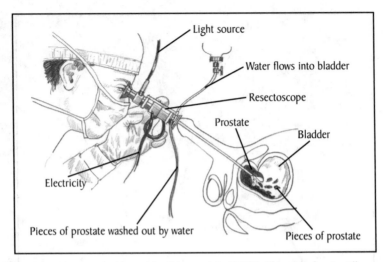

Figure 5.2 - A transurethral resection of the prostate (TURP). This procedure is still considered the "gold standard" of BPH surgical treatment.

Keep tabs on PSA levels

After TURP, your PSA level will fall. During your yearly check for prostate cancer, your doctor may base your PSA levels on your PSA reading after surgery, not your old reading and not what's considered normal for men your age who haven't had TURP.

Transurethral incision of the prostate (TUIP). This procedure is similar to TURP except that instead of removing excess tissue one or two small cuts are made in the prostate to relieve the pressure on the urethra.

This procedure can be done on an outpatient basis, so the hospital stay that TURP usually involves may be avoided. It also has a lower risk of retrograde ejaculation. Other benefits include lower cost, speedier recovery, and better odds for a successful outcome. In addition, the success rates for TURP and TUIP are almost identical. Possible complications include infection and narrowing of the urethra.

However, TUIP only works for men with small to medium-sized prostates (weighs 30 grams or less). If you've definitely decided on surgery, ask your doctor if you're a candidate for TUIP. According to the Agency for Health Care Policy and Research (AHCPR), more men could benefit from this surgery than are currently having it.

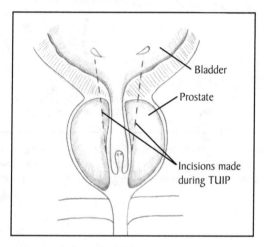

Figure 5.3 - During a transurethral incision of the prostate (TUIP), the surgeon will either make one incision at the 6 o'clock position or two incisions at the 5 o'clock and 7 o'clock positions to relieve pressure on the urethra. Here the surgeon has opted to make two cuts.

Open prostatectomy. This type of surgery is usually reserved for men who have very large prostates that make performing TURP or TUIP unsafe. An open prostatectomy involves making an incision in the lower part of the stomach area and removing the prostate through the bladder or cutting directly into the prostate itself.

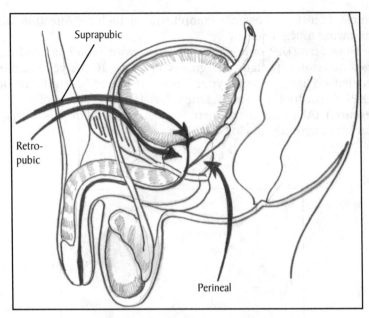

Figure 5.4 - For an open prostatectomy, the surgeon has three possible options for approaching the prostate — the retropubic, suprápubic, or perineal approach. However, the perineal approach is usually only used during a prostatectomy for prostate cancer.

Some doctors think an open prostatectomy may provide longer-lasting benefits than TURP. However, an open prostatectomy has a slightly higher chance of serious complications, like heart attack, pneumonia, or blood clots, because it is a more extensive operation. Also, the recovery period following this surgery is longer than with TURP.

Types of open prostatectomy:

- retropubic — The surgeon goes through your abdominal area to get to your prostate.

- suprapubic — The surgeon goes through your bladder to reach your prostate.

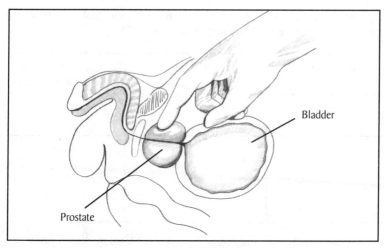

Figure 5.5 - Open prostatectomy: the retropubic approach. In an open prostatectomy, the surgeon makes an incision in the lower part of the stomach area. He will then either remove prostate tissue through the bladder (the suprapubic approach) or cut directly into the prostate itself (the retropubic approach).

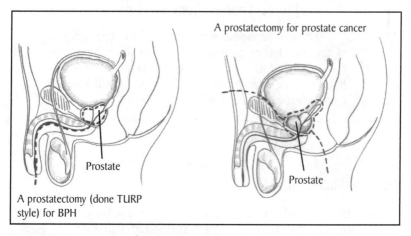

Figure 5.6 - A prostatectomy for BPH is quite different from a prostatectomy for prostate cancer. A prostatectomy for BPH removes all the tissue inside the prostate, leaving only the prostatic capsule. It's like a sack with no groceries inside. A prostatectomy for prostate cancer removes the entire prostate. You have neither sack nor groceries left. The dotted lines show what is removed in each procedure.

The chart below gives you a quick overview of the pros and cons of the most common surgeries for BPH.

Treatment	Chances of symptom improvement	Risk of dying within 3 months of treatment
TURP	85%	2%
TUIP	73%	0.4%
Open prostatectomy	79%	2.6%

1. Calculated from Medicare data years (1988 to 89, Parts A and B), drug cost estimates from drug companies in seven states, and device cost estimates from materials supplied by product manufacturers.

Protect yourself from infection

According to various reports, about 5 to 10 percent of the men having surgery for BPH require a blood transfusion, which always carries a risk of possible infection. See Chapter 6 on ways to reduce your risk of infection from a blood transfusion.

Balloon dilation: It's a bust

The latest word on balloon dilation — it's a bust.

During the 1980s, researchers generated considerable excitement over a promising new technique for treating BPH. An uninflated balloon was placed inside the part of the urethra that lies within the prostate (the prostatic urethra). The balloon was then inflated, pushing away tissue that was putting pressure on the urethra.

Risk of complications	Total incontinence	Hospital stay	Loss of work time	Cost (1,2)
11.9%	1.0%	3-5	7-21 days	$8,606.00 days
17.4%	0.1%	1-3 days	7-21 days	—
24.5% prostatectomy	0.5%	5-10 days	21-28 days	$12,788.00

2. Included in cost estimates for first year after treatment are cost of failure (re-treatment with TURP) and cost of complications following surgery, such as incontinence, narrowing of the urethra, or shrinking of the bladder neck.

— No data available.

Actually, balloon dilation is not really new at all. It's just a new version of the old technique of prostate dilation, which has been around for centuries. Early attempts at dilation involved a variety of tools but never a balloon.

At first, success with dilation was limited by problems in reaching the prostatic urethra. It wasn't until the 1950s that researchers invented a special metal tool designed to expand once it was inside the prostate. This made both reaching and expanding the constricted urethra much easier. In the 1980s, researchers suggested using a balloon as the dilator instead of the old metal tool. Balloon dilation was just a new twist on an old technique.

Unfortunately, the new twist has not made this treatment any more effective for treating BPH. The most recent studies show no long-term improvements, and the procedure is no longer generally recommended. In fact, manufacturers have stopped making the balloons, and most insurance companies no longer offer reimbursement for this procedure.

The best and brightest of future treatments

Although several of the following treatments are used fairly regularly by some doctors to treat BPH, most researchers feel that not enough studies have been completed on the new procedures to determine their effectiveness. Still, if your doctor offers you one of these therapies, you may want to seriously consider giving it a try. Many of them are less invasive than the traditional therapies and have fewer complications as well. However, before you decide to go ahead, make sure your insurance company will pay for a treatment that may be considered experimental.

If your insurance won't cover it, ask your doctor about participating in a clinical trial. If you have access to a computer that connects to the World Wide Web, you can also check a site called CenterWatch, which is a clinical trials listing service. Their Internet address is http://www.centerwatch.com/.

Clinical trials almost always cover all the costs of treatment. Researchers use clinical trials to find out if promising new treatment methods really work. If you participate in one of these treatment studies, you will be given the new treatment and carefully watched. All your reactions will be noted and compared with others.

Transurethral microwave thermotherapy (TUMT). Several new treatments have the potential to make the undesirable side effects of traditional surgery a thing of the past. One of the devices used to deliver a type of heat therapy called transurethral microwave therapy (TUMT) recently received approval by the FDA.

Dubbed the Prostatron, this computer-controlled device uses microwaves to heat and destroy excess prostate tissue. Both safe and effective, TUMT has two added bonuses many men find very appealing. It usually does not lead to sexual difficulties or incontinence.

During treatment, a flexible plastic catheter containing a small microwave antenna is placed into the urethra and positioned as close to the enlarged prostate as possible. Once in position, the Prostatron machine is turned on and directs microwave energy into the prostate. Targeted portions of the prostate are heated to at least 111 degrees Fahrenheit. A cooling system protects the urinary tract during the procedure.

Tested on 375 men over age 45 at seven medical centers in the United States, this device relieved urgency, frequency, straining, and start-and-stop urination in 75 percent of the men. For half of the men, TUMT continued to provide relief four years after treatment.

For the other half, it was a different story. They either required re-treatment, drugs, or surgery during that time. In addition, the procedure did not improve a weak urinary stream or incomplete emptying of the bladder. The most common complication was urinary retention. This problem typically develops within 12 hours of treatment. However, retention has occurred as late as two to four days following the procedure. Usually, a catheter used for one to two weeks will resolve the problem. Other possible side effects include bladder spasms and bleeding.

TUMT takes about one hour. It can be done on an outpatient basis using only a local anesthetic. Because of the device's design, it can only be used in men with medium-sized prostates. Also, it may take six weeks to three months for changes to become significantly noticeable.

High intensity focused ultrasound (HIFU). This method works much like TUMT, but it may be able to focus energy directly on the area that needs to be destroyed, sparing the surrounding healthy tissue. However, it usually causes temporary urinary retention and blood in the semen. Also, long-term effects are not known, and researchers suspect it may not be very effective in men with large prostate glands.

Transurethral needle ablation (TUNA). Also a type of heat therapy, TUNA uses radio frequency energy to destroy excess prostate tissue. A rigid catheter with a telescope inside is inserted into the urethra. Using the telescope to guide him, the urologist pushes needles that emit radio frequency energy through the catheter and into the prostate where it destroys excess prostate tissue. Approved by the FDA in 1996, TUNA usually takes about an hour and can be done on an outpatient basis.

TUNA seems to work best in men who have slight obstructions. It doesn't appear to be as effective as more traditional treatments in relieving symptoms and increasing urine flow. However, no one knows what the long-term benefits of TUNA may be. Side effects may include temporary urine retention or bloody urine, urinary tract infection, or retrograde ejaculation.

Visual laser ablation of the prostate (VLAP). This is one of the new laser treatments currently being tested. The surgeon performing VLAP uses a piece of equipment that combines a laser and a tiny camera. The picture is projected on a television monitor. This lets the doctor see exactly how to direct the laser beam.

If ultrasound is used to direct placement of the laser fibers, the procedure is often called ILCP, which stands for Interstitial Laser Coagulation of the Prostate. Another procedure called Clap or Contact Visual Laser Ablation of the Prostate involves direct contact of the laser fibers to the prostate tissue, using a tiny camera for guidance.

The high temperatures kill the extra prostate tissue, which is gradually shed by the prostate over the next couple of weeks and is either absorbed by the body or washed away in the urine.

Benefits include a shorter time spent in surgery, less trauma, faster recovery time, and less risk of bleeding. However, this technique produces irritating symptoms for a fairly long time after treatment. In addition, a longer period of catheterization is needed, and it may be six to eight weeks before you notice any improvement.

Transurethral vaporization of the prostate (TVP). This procedure is similar to TURP, but instead of cutting away excess tissue, an electric current vaporizes the extra tissue. (The tissue actually

Determine the treatment that's right for you

Treatment	Pros
TURP	Can sometimes be done on an outpatient basis, although usually requires a short hospital stay. Quick recovery, effectively relieves symptoms.
TUIP	Can be done on outpatient basis. Lower cost, speedier recovery, better odds for a successful outcome. Lower risk of retrograde ejaculation.

turns to steam.) TVP involves a shorter hospital stay and perhaps less risk of bleeding, incontinence, or narrowing of the urethra.

Hot new surgical cure

Many laser surgeries are done with the neodynium:yttrium aluminum garnet laser, abbreviated Nd:YAG. This laser can produce temperatures between 932 and 1,292 degrees Fahrenheit. To put these numbers in perspective, consider that your normal body temperature is about 98.6 degrees Fahrenheit.

Stents. A stent is a plastic or metal device that is inserted through the urethra to the narrowed area and allowed to expand, like a spring. Stents can be inserted quickly, require little recovery time, do not affect sexual functioning, and may eliminate the need for a catheter. On the downside, they may cause frequent or painful urination for days or weeks following the procedure.

Usually, these devices are only used on older men. Stents are also an option for men who are not good candidates for more extensive surgery or for men who require a temporary treatment.

Cons	Complications
Will have to wear a catheter for 12 to 36 hours after surgery.	Bleeding, infection, narrowing of the urethra, impotence, incontinence, retrograde ejaculation.
Only works on men with small to medium-sized prostates.	Infection, narrowing of the urethra.

Determine the treatment that's right for you (continued)

Treatment	Pros
Open prostatectomy	Offers longer lasting relief to men with large prostates. May have fewer long-term complications.
TUMT	Can be done on an outpatient basis. Takes only about one hour. Does not cause blood loss or lead to impotence or incontinence.
HIFU	Spares healthy parts of prostate while getting rid of excess tissue.
TUNA	Treatment only takes about an hour. Can be done on outpatient basis.
Laser prostatectomy (VLAP, ILCP, CLAP)	Shorter time in surgery, less trauma, faster recovery time, less risk of bleeding.
TVP	Involves shorter hospital stay and less risk of bleeding, incontinence, or narrowing of the urethra.
Stents	Can be inserted quickly, require little recovery time, do not affect sexual functioning, may eliminate the need for a catheter. Good option for older men who are not good candidates for more extensive surgery.

Cons	Complications
Slightly higher risk of serious complications.	Blood clot, heart attack, pneumonia.
May require use of a catheter for a week or so. Also, may be difficult to find a doctor trained in this procedure.	Urinary retention, bleeding, bladder spasms, blood in the semen.
Long-term effects not known. Also, may not be that effective in men with large prostate glands. In addition, this procedure is rarely performed in North America.	Blood in the urine or semen, temporary urinary retention
Seems to work best in men who have only slight obstructions. Not as effective as more traditional treatments in relieving symptoms and increasing urine flow.	Temporary urine retention or bloody urine, urinary tract infection, retrograde ejaculation.
May be six to eight weeks before you notice any improvement, requires longer period wearing a catheter.	Irritating symptoms may persist for a long time following treatment.
May not remove as much excess tissue as some other procedures.	Irritating symptoms may persist for a long time following treatment.
Long-term effects not known. May cause more urinary tract infections.	May cause frequent or painful urination for days or weeks.

Optional tests may optimize your outcome

Uroflow test. Although the uroflow test is not required to diagnose BPH, you may want to discuss this diagnostic tool with your doctor. Some studies show that men who are evaluated with the uroflow test have higher surgery success rates than men who do not have this test, even though many urologists think this test is unnecessary.

The apparent reason for the improved rate of success is that one-third of men who are told they have BPH (making them potential candidates for surgery) are actually found to have some other problem when this test is done. This test will clarify if your problems are indeed caused by an enlarged prostate or by something else.

Naturally, if you have surgery for BPH when your problems are caused by something else entirely, you're not very likely to experience any benefit at all.

Uroflowmetry, another name for the uroflow test, is simple and painless. All you need is a full bladder. You urinate into a special toilet, which measures how much urine you pass and records the speed of your urine stream.

After completing the uroflow test, your doctor may also have you take the residual urine test. This procedure is designed to show if the bladder empties normally or not. A catheter is inserted into the bladder to empty and measure any remaining urine.

Other optional tests your doctor may suggest before surgery include the following.

Pressure flow studies. If the uroflow test suggests you do not have an obstruction, this study will confirm whether or not you will benefit from surgery. This test measures the pressure in your bladder as you urinate. That number is then compared to the speed of your urine stream. Some doctors feel this test is the best way to find out how much your ability to urinate is affected.

For example, some men may have strong urine streams even though they have significant obstruction from BPH just because they can generate high bladder pressure. These men could benefit from treatment to relieve their obstructions although the uroflow test might suggest otherwise. Pressure flow studies can also reveal if a low urinary flow rate is caused by a diseased bladder, in which case treatment for obstruction would not be much help.

In the pressure flow study, a small tube called a catheter is inserted into your penis, through the urethra, and into your bladder. The test may cause discomfort for a short time. In a few men, it may cause a urinary tract infection.

Urethrocystoscopy. This is a helpful test for your doctor to perform before surgery as it can point out any problems in your urethra and bladder before your doctor actually goes digging around in your prostate. Using a special tool inserted through the penis tip and up into the urethra, your doctor can examine your entire urethra for other complications that may be causing your urination problems, such as narrowing of the urethra called urethral stricture. This knowledge helps your doctor determine the best treatment approach.

For more practical tips on what you can do to prepare your body for surgery, see Chapter 6.

5 tips for successful recovery

After surgery, you will probably notice some blood or clots in your urine as the wound starts to heal. If your bladder is being irrigated (flushed with water), you may notice that your urine becomes red once the irrigation is stopped. Some bleeding is normal, but it should clear up by the time you leave the hospital.

Take it easy the first few weeks after you get home. You may not have any pain, but you still have an incision that is healing — even with transurethral surgery where the incision can't be seen.

Since many people try to do too much after surgery and then have a setback, it's a good idea to talk to your doctor before resuming your normal routine. During this initial period of recovery at home, avoid any straining or sudden movements that could tear your incision. Here are some guidelines:

- Drink at least eight cups of water a day to help flush out your bladder and speed healing.

- Avoid straining during bowel movements. Eat foods high in fiber, like whole grains, vegetables, and fruit, to prevent constipation. Take a laxative if you become constipated.

- Lay off the heavy lifting.

- Don't drive or operate machinery.

- Avoid sex (ejaculation) for several weeks.

See Chapter 6 for more suggestions on how to make a healthy and rapid recovery after surgery.

Complications of surgery

Complications of prostate surgery range from infection to pneumonia to stroke, but most complications are fairly uncommon.

Sometimes scar tissue resulting from surgery requires treatment a year or so after surgery. Rarely, the opening of the bladder becomes scarred and shrinks, causing obstruction. This problem may require a surgical procedure similar to transurethral incision. More often, scar tissue may form in the urethra and cause narrowing. The doctor can usually solve this problem during an office visit by stretching the urethra.

See Chapter 6 for more tips on dealing with possible complications.

Small setbacks that are part of your recovery

Even though you'll probably feel much better by the time you leave the hospital, it could take a couple of months for you to heal completely. Here are some of the problems you're likely to encounter on the road to recovery.

Problems urinating. You may notice that your urine stream is stronger right after surgery, but it may take awhile before you can urinate normally again. After the catheter is removed, urine will pass over the surgical wound on the prostate, and you may initially have some discomfort or feel a sense of urgency when you urinate. This problem will gradually go away. After a couple of months, you should be able to urinate less often and more easily.

Incontinence. As your bladder returns to normal, you may have some temporary problems controlling urination, but long-term incontinence rarely occurs. Doctors find that the longer problems existed before surgery, the longer it will take for the bladder to regain its full function after the operation. For more information on dealing with incontinence, see Chapter 12.

Bleeding. In the first few weeks after transurethral surgery, the scab inside the bladder may loosen, and blood may suddenly appear in the urine. Although this can be alarming, the bleeding usually stops after a short period of bed rest and drinking lots of liquids. However, if your urine is so red it is difficult to see through or it contains clots, call your doctor. If you are having any discomfort, make sure you let him know.

Rekindling the romance

What does surgery mean for your sex life? Experts aren't exactly sure. Some say it rarely affects sexual function, while others say it causes problems in 30 percent of all men who have surgery.

Many doctors have found that, although it takes awhile for sexual function to return fully, most men are able to enjoy sex again. However, complete recovery of sexual function may take up to one year. The exact length of time depends on how long BPH surgery was postponed despite symptoms and on the type of surgery done. Basically, here's how surgery is likely to affect the following aspects of your sexuality.

Erections. Most doctors agree that if you were able to have an erection before surgery, you'll probably be able to do so after surgery. However, if you weren't able to have an erection before surgery, don't expect a major miracle in that department now.

Ejaculation. After surgery, many men experience retrograde ejaculation. Although retrograde ejaculation renders most men sterile, your doctor can retrieve sperm from your bladder and use them to artificially inseminate your mate so you may still be able to father a child.

Orgasm. You should still be able to enjoy sex as much after surgery as before, although the sensation of retrograde ejaculation may take a little getting used to. Actually, any concerns you have about sex can interfere with your performance and enjoyment of it as much as the surgery itself. That's why it's so important to discuss any worries with your doctor. Many men also find it helpful to talk to a counselor during the adjustment period after surgery.

Fend off future problems

In the years after surgery, it's important to continue to have regular checkups and rectal exams. Also, be sure to report any suspicious symptoms to your doctor.

Since surgery for BPH leaves a good part of the gland behind, it's still possible for prostate problems to pop up, including cancer. However, surgery usually offers relief from BPH for at least 15 years. Of the men who have surgery for BPH, 15 to 20 percent eventually will need a second operation. One possible reason for a second surgery is that the prostate grows back. Also, some men require another surgery if the first operation causes a scar to form, which blocks the urinary tract.

In summary

Most men with BPH prefer to save surgery as their last option. Although surgery may offer the most relief from your symptoms, it can also have the most serious side effects, including impotence, incontinence, retrograde ejaculation, and even death. Generally, men bothered by severe symptoms of BPH benefit most from surgery.

Don't agree to surgery simply because your doctor says your symptoms will get worse. The truth is that BPH symptoms progress slowly and even improve spontaneously in some cases.

However, some men don't have a choice. If you have a stubborn case of urinary retention that won't respond to catheter treatment, recurring urinary tract infections, urine that is frequently bloody, bladder stones, or kidney problems caused by BPH, most doctors will strongly recommend surgery as being in the best interest of your health.

If you've definitely decided on surgery to treat your BPH, you have a number of options to choose from. Among the more traditional, extensively tested options for BPH, you have three choices:

▶ **Transurethral prostatectomy (TURP).** Traditionally, the "gold standard" for treating BPH, TURP involves going through your urethra to reach the prostate and cutting away excess prostate tissue.

▶ **Transurethral incision of the prostate (TUIP).** This procedure is similar to TURP except that instead of removing excess tissue, one or two small cuts are made in the prostate to relieve pressure on the urethra. This procedure also involves going through the urethra to reach the prostate.

Success rates for TURP and TUIP are almost identical. Other benefits of TUIP include lower cost, speedier recovery, and better odds for a successful outcome. Ask your doctor if you're a good candidate for TUIP (your prostate needs to weigh 30 grams or less).

▶ **Open prostatectomy.** This surgery involves making an incision in the lower part of the stomach area and removing the prostate through the bladder or cutting directly into the prostate itself. This surgery is usually reserved for men who have very large prostates, which makes performing TURP or TUIP unsafe.

The chart on page 108 gives you a quick overview of the pros and cons for the most traditional BPH treatments.

Although only three traditional treatments are available for relieving the symptoms of BPH, a large number of up-and-coming treatments for BPH greatly expand your choices. However, some of these techniques are still considered experimental. In addition to possibly less reliable results from these treatments, you may have trouble getting your insurance company to pay for them. That doesn't mean you shouldn't consider them. You may be able to cover the cost of the procedure by participating in a clinical trial. Your doctor should be able to help you track down that information.

Some men opt to pay for new procedures out of their own pockets if it seems to be their best option. See page 10 for a complete description of these up-and-coming treatments, as well as a chart comparing the pros, cons, and complications of each type of procedure. Work with your doctor in choosing the treatment that is best for you.

Once you've made your decision, it's time to prepare for the big day. You and your doctor may decide that it's in your best interest to undergo a few optional tests. These tests can help your doctor decide the best treatment approach for you.

Once surgery is over, you only have a few more hurdles before you're home free. First and foremost, you want to do everything you can to avoid post-surgery complications. See Chapter 6 for more suggestions on avoiding complications of all sorts.

Typically, you'll also have a few problems urinating or controlling urination (incontinence) after surgery. You may also spot some blood in your urine. Don't panic. Most of these problems are perfectly normal and will disappear with time. However, be sure you report all problems to your doctor. He can give you some helpful tips about how to handle these situations.

You will probably also experience some difficulty with sex after surgery. The good news is that most men regain their sexual functions, although it may take up to a year. The bad news is that if you had problems with sex before surgery, you shouldn't expect a miracle now.

Surgery for BPH usually offers symptom relief for at least 15 years. However, since most surgeries leave much of your prostate in place, it's still possible for problems to pop up. That's why it's important to get yearly checkups and report any unusual symptoms to your doctor immediately.

I've developed a new philosophy ...
I only dread one day at a time.
Charlie Brown, comic strip character
by cartoonist Charles Schultz

Don't be afraid to take a big step if one is indicated;
you can't cross a chasm in two small jumps.
David Lloyd George, Prime Minister of England
during World War I

6

Surgery: Before and after

Before your surgery

7 tips you need to know

No matter what kind of surgery you're having, there are some things you need to know to make your surgery a success:

▶ Ask if there are different ways of doing the surgery you're scheduled for. Some methods involve more extensive operations than others. Ask your doctor why he chose his method.

▶ Find out where you'll have your surgery. Most surgeons use one or two local hospitals. Ask your doctor if he knows how many operations like the one you're scheduled for have been performed in that hospital. If he doesn't know, call the hospital administration office and ask. Also ask about the hospital's success rates with this particular operation. The reason for making this extra effort is that some hospitals have higher success rates in certain operations than others. You want to use the hospital with the best success rate. However, some surgeries are now done on an outpatient basis, either in the doctor's office or in a special day surgery unit. If your doctor says you'll be having surgery as an outpatient, ask if that surgery is normally done on an outpatient basis. If not, ask why you'll be undergoing that surgery as an outpatient. You want to be in the right place for your operation.

▶ Have your doctor completely and clearly explain the surgery. Ask him what will happen to you before, during, and after your operation. Find out what kind of supplies, equipment, or any other help you'll need after surgery. Knowing exactly what to expect will help calm your fears and worries. Generally, the fewer anxieties and worries you have, the faster your body will heal.

▶ Ask your doctor about taking aspirin and any medicines that contain aspirin. Most of the time, your doctor will want you to stop taking these drugs at least a week before surgery. You should also ask your doctor what he wants you to do about other medicines you take regularly. Finally, let your doctor know if you drink or smoke regularly because these habits can affect the anesthesia.

▶ Don't eat or drink anything after midnight the night before your surgery. This is the general rule for people having surgery, but check with your doctor just in case. Some people are allowed to have clear liquids up to a few hours before they receive anesthesia.

▶ Arrange for a responsible adult to take you home after your surgery. Unless your surgery involves only local anesthesia (see *What to expect from anesthesia* later in this chapter for an explanation of local anesthesia), you won't be allowed to drive yourself home.

▶ Dress for comfort. Wear loose-fitting clothes and leave your valuables at home.

Top 10 hospitals in the United States

Just like doctors, some hospitals rate better than others. It's usually in your best interest to get treatment at the best hospital you can find. The more serious the problem, the better the hospital you'll want to be in. According to *U.S. News and World Report*, these are the best hospitals in the United States for treating urologically related problems.

A brief description of the different categories will help you better understand the rankings.

"U.S. News Index" is an overall measurement of the hospital's quality of care. One-third of the score comes from the "reputational score," one-third from the "mortality rate," and the final third comes from urology data, including use of advanced medical technology and the types of services available to patients with special needs. The top hospital receives a score of 100.

"Reputational score" is the percentage of board-certified urologists surveyed in 1995, 1996, and 1997 who named the hospital among the top five. Results from 1995, 1996, and 1997 are pooled.

"Urology mortality rate" compares the actual number of deaths to the expected number. The lower the mortality rate, the better.

"COTH member" indicates membership in the elite Council of Teaching Hospitals.

"Technology score" reflects the availability of urology-related medical technology.

"Urology discharges" is the number of medical and surgical discharges from the hospital reported to the federal government in 1994 and 1995. Higher is better as quality usually rises with volume.

"RNs to beds" is hospitalwide ratio of full-time registered nurses to beds over a 24-hour period. During a regular eight-hour shift, the number of nurses to beds is about one-third of the number shown. Higher is better.

"Trauma center" indicates whether on-site trauma services are offered.

Top 10 hospitals in the United States for treating urologically related problems

Rank	Hospital	U.S. News Index	Reputational Score	Urology Mortality Rate
1	Johns Hopkins Hospital Baltimore	100.0	55.7%	1.59
2	Mayo Clinic Rochester, Minn.	76.3	37.8%	0.27
3	UCLA Medical Center Los Angeles	50.2	22.9%	1.00
4	Massachusetts General Hospital, Boston	46.7	20.4%	1.01
5	Cleveland Clinic	45.1	19.3%	0.47
6	Duke University Medical Center, Durham, N.C.	38.5	14.5%	0.65
7	Barnes-Jewish Hospital St. Louis	35.2	15.2%	1.02
8	Stanford University Hospital, Stanford, Conn.	35.1	12.8%	0.50
9	Baylor University Medical Center, Dallas	30.4	10.2%	0.90
10	Memorial Sloan-Kettering Cancer Center, New York	29.1	8.9%	0.60

How you can help guarantee good results

Not only is the skill of your surgeon and your hospital's success rate important to the outcome of your surgery, how you prepare your body plays a big part, too.

COTH Member	Technology Score (of 8)	Urology Discharges	RNs to Beds	Trauma Center
Yes	8.0	763	1.32	Yes
Yes	7.0	2,449	1.52	Yes
Yes	8.0	939	1.25	Yes
Yes	8.0	1,184	1.66	Yes
Yes	7.5	1,177	1.06	No
Yes	8.0	1,175	1.60	No
Yes	8.0	1,028	0.77	No
Yes	6.0	702	1.09	Yes
Yes	7.0	925	1.52	Yes
Yes	7.0	1,084	1.52	No

"A calm, rested, well-nourished, fit patient does better every time," says Dr. J. Curtis Nickel, professor of urology at Queens University in Kingston, Ontario. He offers these tips to help you prepare your body.

▶ **Exercise.** Regular exercise will improve your circulation and help your heart and lungs prepare for the shock of surgery. It will also help your body make the best use of the nutrients from your food. Dr. Nickel's exercise of choice: walking.

▶ **Eat a well-balanced diet.** This prepares your body tissues for the healing process. If you're overweight and having surgery by choice, instead of emergency surgery, consider taking off a few pounds before you schedule your operation. The closer you are to a normal weight, the less likely you are to have problems with anesthesia. You'll also heal better and be less likely to have complications after surgery. Before you start any weight loss program, especially if you may need to have surgery fairly soon, talk with your doctor.

▶ **Rest.** It's important that you don't tire yourself out before surgery. Also, try to avoid stressful or anxiety-provoking situations before surgery.

▶ **Consider vitamin supplements.** Taking a multivitamin prior to surgery may aid the healing process.

What to expect from anesthesia

Surgeons use anesthesia so they can perform surgery without causing you unnecessary pain. Your doctor will be able to tell you whether your operation calls for local, regional, or general anesthesia.

Local anesthesia only numbs a specific part of your body for a short period of time. Regional anesthesia numbs a larger part of your body — for example, the lower half — for a few hours. With both local and regional anesthesia, you will be awake for your operation unless you ask to be given something that will cause you to go to sleep. With general anesthesia, which knocks you out completely, your entire body will be numb during surgery.

Although anesthesia may seem a little scary, it's a lot less scary than having surgery without it. Also, anesthesia is almost completely safe for most people. Either an anesthesiologist (a doctor who specializes in anesthesia) or a nurse anesthetist will be responsible for your anesthesia. Both are highly skilled and specially trained in this field.

It's a good idea to meet the person who will be responsible for your anesthesia before you have surgery. This will give the anesthesiologist a chance to become familiar with your complete medical history, examine you carefully, and find out what medicines you're currently taking. He can discuss your anesthesia options with you, as well as explain the risks and benefits of your different choices. Although your doctor and anesthesiologist will take your desires into consideration, they make the final choice about what type of anesthesia is best for you.

Side effects from anesthesia may include drowsiness, muscle aches, sore throat, dizziness, headaches, and nausea. Although side effects normally wear off fairly quickly after surgery, it may take several days for them to disappear completely.

If your surgery involves only a short stay at the hospital (a day or less), it's important to remember that for 24 hours after anesthesia, you should not drink alcohol or take nonprescription medicines, drive a car or operate heavy machinery, or make important decisions.

How to avoid a blood transfusion tragedy

Although the risk of a transfusion infection is probably lower than it's ever been due to the increased safety of the blood supply, there's no such thing as a totally risk-free transfusion. Some types of hepatitis are still not detectable with blood tests. Also, there is a period of time when a blood test won't show that someone is infected with HIV. During this time, a person with unknown HIV could easily pass it on through blood donation. In addition, there may be other deadly viruses floating around out there that have yet to be identified.

As if that's not enough, some research also suggests that blood transfusions may suppress the immune system. If you have a transfusion during surgery, that could slow down your healing process — even making you more likely to develop wound infections.

What all this scary stuff adds up to is that you should not have a blood transfusion unless it's absolutely essential. Studies suggest that up to 55 percent of blood transfusions may be unnecessary.

Just to be on the safe side, you may want to consider donating two pints of blood for your own use before surgery, especially if your surgeon expects a particularly difficult operation. However, it will take several weeks after a donation for your body to recover. Ask your doctor about donating blood long before your surgery. If your doctor says a blood transfusion is likely and you can't donate blood for yourself or don't have enough blood donated to cover your needs, ask your doctor to keep the amount you receive to a minimum. It is also sometimes possible for the doctor to filter and transfuse your own blood during the operation. The bottom line: The more blood you get that isn't yours, the greater your risk of infection.

Protect yourself from a medical hex

Although a medical hex may sound like hocus pocus, research suggests such a thing may be possible.

It's true that modern doctors don't go around hexing people in the same way that witch doctors and voodoo priests are famous for. However, Dr. Larry Dossey, author of *Be Careful What You Pray For ... You Just Might Get It*, suggests that what is said while you're under anesthesia can have a similar effect.

Researchers have known for years that even under complete anesthesia people still continue to hear. Even people given regional anesthesia along with a drug to make them sleepy can hear what's going on around them. Unfortunately, doctors doing surgery may not always keep this important point in mind. In some cases, a surgeon or even his assistants' casual comments may be a matter of life or death to the patient.

Dr. Dossey uses the example of a young man undergoing surgery for a hernia to illustrate this point. During the surgery, a first-year medical student jokingly commented, "This is the worst case I have ever seen." He simply meant it was the worst case he'd ever seen because it was the only case he'd ever seen.

However, to the young man undergoing surgery who overheard the comment, the effect was much more serious. After the surgeon completed what he considered a routine operation, the young man's condition continued to deteriorate. He confessed to a nurse that he fully expected to die. Finally, after the young man had consulted with a psychiatrist and undergone hypnosis, the doctor discovered the root of the problem — the medical student's joking comment.

Once the medical student explained to the young man that his comment had been nothing more than a bad joke, the patient made a full recovery.

To protect yourself from possible medical hexing during surgery, Dossey offers these suggestions.

- Discuss your concerns with your surgeon and anesthesiologist. Knowing how you feel may encourage them to keep their comments positive and upbeat.

- Consider listening to tapes of your own choice during surgery. You may want to make your own tape of positive, encouraging comments or simply listen to a musical selection you enjoy. Some hospitals have a variety of tapes to choose from.

The best way to avoid medical hexing is to go into the procedure with a positive, hopeful, upbeat attitude. If you truly believe your surgery will be a success, there's a much greater chance that it will be.

6 steps to effective pain management

Ask your doctor what to expect after surgery. Being prepared helps put you in control and lessens anxiety, which can actually make pain worse. Here are some good questions to ask:

- Will there be much pain after surgery?

- Where will I hurt?

- How long will the pain last?

Discuss your pain control options before surgery. Your pain relief options include taking painkillers before, during, and after surgery. Discuss with your doctor which plan will be most helpful for you.

You'll make it easier for your doctor to guide you in a pain relief plan if you tell him which pain relief methods worked or didn't work for you in the past. Be sure to let your doctor know which over-the-counter and prescription drugs you are currently taking. Also, tell him about any allergies you may have. This is also a good time to discuss any concerns you have about pain medicines, such as possible side effects.

Talk about your pain management schedule in the hospital. Some people get pain medicines in the hospital only when they ask for them. Sometimes, there are delays, and the pain just gets worse while they wait. Here are two ways you can avoid those potentially painful problems:

▶ Ask that your pain pills or shots be given at set times. Instead of waiting until you can't stand it any more, you receive medicine at set times during the day to keep pain under control. If you are scheduled for an open prostatectomy, ask your anesthesiologist to use an epidural catheter for drug relief during the first day or so after your operation. The epidural catheter provides excellent pain relief for the open prostatectomy.

▶ Put a request in for patient-controlled analgesia (PCA). With PCA, you control when you get pain medicine. When you begin to feel pain, you press a button to inject the medicine through the intravenous (IV) tube in your arm.

Don't be a silent sufferer. When it comes to pain after surgery, don't worry about being a bother. You need to tell your nurse or doctor about pain you have because it can signal a problem with your operation.

Relax your way to pain relief. Simple relaxation techniques, such as abdominal breathing, can increase your comfort after surgery. To enjoy the relaxing effects of abdominal breathing, simply inhale and exhale slowly.

To make sure you're breathing for maximum benefit, look at your stomach. As you breathe in and out, it should move up and down. Your chest should stay still. Whether you have a few seconds or half an hour, a little abdominal breathing can stop stress and control anxiety, both of which can worsen pain.

Put a lid on your pain with nifty nondrug solutions. Massage, hot and cold packs, music, and positive thinking can all work little mini-miracles when it comes to relieving pain. Experiment to see which works best for you.

Some hospitals also offer a rather unusual pain relief option called transcutaneous electrical nerve stimulation (TENS). Using mild electrical stimulation on your skin, this system provides nondrug relief by interfering with pain's pathway to your brain. By stopping your brain from registering the pain, you don't have any discomfort.

Beta blocker reduces heart complications

If you're scheduled for prostate surgery and you're worried about how your heart will hold up, consider asking your doctor about atenolol.

About 3 million of the 30 million people who undergo surgery every year have heart problems that make surgery a greater risk. These problems can increase the risk of serious complications, including death, two to 20 times during the two years after surgery. Problems seem to be linked to an increased heart rate caused by the anxiety of being in the hospital.

The good news is that the beta-blocking drug atenolol may be able to reduce the number of heart complications and deaths for as long as two years after surgery, according to a recent study in *The New England Journal of Medicine*. In one group of patients, atenolol was given intravenously before surgery and immediately afterward. After that, it was taken by mouth for the remainder of the hospital stay. The other group of patients received only a placebo (a fake pill or treatment). After two years, survival rates were 83 percent for the atenolol group but only 68 percent for the placebo group.

This study suggests that atenolol may be a good option for men who need prostate surgery but have heart disease or are at risk of heart disease. However, experts stress that atenolol is only indicated for some people at high risk of heart disease. It could be dangerous for other people.

After your surgery

Give yourself permission to control your pain

It used to be that people thought pain was a necessary part of having surgery. Today, that's no longer true. These days, you can work with your nurses and doctors before and after surgery to prevent or relieve pain. Pain control can help you in three important ways:

- **Boost your comfort level.** Controlling pain will make you more comfortable as your body heals.

- **Heal your body faster.** With less pain, you can start walking, do your breathing exercises, and get your strength back more quickly. You may even leave the hospital sooner.

- **Improve your results.** People whose pain is well-controlled seem to do better after surgery. They also may avoid problems such as pneumonia and blood clots that affect others.

Stop pain before it starts

Don't try to be a long-suffering super-hero after surgery. You'll live to regret it, but you may wish you hadn't.

One of the most common mistakes people make during hospital stays is waiting until they are in severe pain before asking for pain relief. It's very rare to become addicted to a painkiller during a short hospital stay. Besides, nurses say, it takes more medicine to relieve pain than to prevent it.

Most pain medicines are listed on your chart as PRN (pro re nata). That's Latin for "as needed." You have to ask for it before you get it. However, the nurse will usually give you your medicine on a regular schedule, every four hours or so, if you make it clear that's what you'd prefer. Or, you can ask for your medicine 20 minutes before you think you'll really need it.

Even better, ask for PCA (Patient Controlled Analgesia). With this handy system, you can give the pain medicine to yourself when you need it by pressing a button to inject the medicine through the intravenous (IV) tube in your vein.

If you aren't getting adequate relief, ask your nurse to see if your doctor can prescribe another painkiller. Medicines have different effects on different people.

Make a rapid recovery

Following surgery, you'll probably stay in the hospital from three to 10 days depending on the type of surgery you had and how quickly you recover.

At the end of surgery, a special catheter is inserted through the opening of the penis to drain urine from the bladder into a collection bag. Called a Foley catheter, this device has a balloon attached at one end. After the catheter is inserted into the bladder, the balloon is filled with sterile water. This prevents the catheter from leaving the bladder until the balloon is emptied.

You'll probably need the catheter for a couple of days. Sometimes, the catheter causes recurring, painful bladder spasms the day after surgery. These may be difficult to control, but they will eventually disappear.

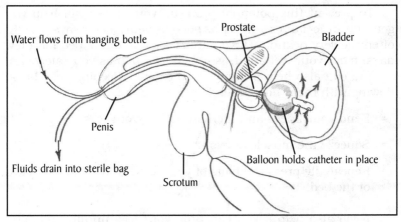

Figure 6.1 - Foley catheter. This device is inserted through the opening of the penis to drain urine from the bladder into a collection bag. It is normally removed a few days after surgery.

How to beat a blood clot

One of the possible complications of prostate surgery, especially an open prostatectomy, is a pulmonary embolism (the medical term for a blood clot that plugs the arteries supplying blood to the lungs).

Surgery itself sets the stage for the development of clots in your lower legs. In most cases, the problem actually starts during surgery. Lying around after surgery increases that risk. Open prostatectomy presents more problems because you typically have to lie around a little longer after this surgery than some of the other types.

Normally, your calf muscles help your blood circulate by squeezing the deep veins in your legs. That helps push the blood back up to your heart. When you're inactive, blood can stagnate in your veins. It thickens and slows down, making clots more likely to form.

About half the people with deep vein blood clots have no symptoms. When symptoms do occur where the clot has formed, they may include slight swelling of the leg or calf, tenderness, cramplike pain, chills, fever, a bluish skin color, and protruding leg veins.

To prevent this potential problem, your nurse will help you get on your feet after surgery as soon as your doctor says it's OK, often the very next day. If you aren't allowed out of bed for a few days, move your feet and legs in bed as much as you safely can.

You can also help prevent blood clots by keeping your blood flowing with these hospital-bed exercises:

- Bend your knees and then straighten your legs.

- Squeeze the muscles in your calves.

- Repeatedly press the balls of your feet against the footboard of the bed.

It will also help if you can prop your legs up after surgery. Most people in the hospital lie with their heads propped up. To reduce the risk of blood clots, lie flat with your legs elevated about 6 inches. This position will get your blood flowing better. It's also recommended after you come home from the hospital. See the following box for more easy exercises that can help you beat a blood clot.

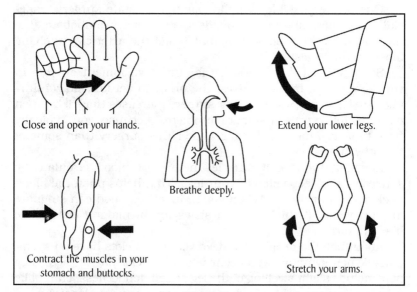

Figure 6.2 - Prevent blood clots with these easy-to-do exercises.

Music encourages healing

As miraculous as it may sound, music, especially Mozart's music, may help you heal faster after surgery.

Since ancient times, people have recognized music as a powerful healing tool. The early Hebrews and Christians believed that singing the Psalms could promote healing. And the Bible records how David's playing of the harp cured King Saul's depression.

New research supports many of the ancient claims about music's healing powers. Scientific studies provide evidence that music can lower blood pressure and heart rate, relieve pain, increase energy, boost intelligence, combat depression, and reduce stress.

In 1979, Helen Bonny, a Baltimore psychotherapist with a doctorate in music and psychology, developed crushing chest pains. The diagnosis — heart disease. During the next few years, Bonny underwent several hospital stays and, finally, coronary bypass surgery.

During these trying times, Bonny used tapes of her favorite music to keep her spirits up. Slowly, as she regained her health, she came to believe that the music had physical healing powers as well. Later, she was able to put her theory to the test in the intensive and coronary care units at St. Agnes Hospital, Baltimore, and Jefferson General Hospital in Port Townsend, Wash.

People in critical care who listened to the tapes Bonny had specially created to promote healing experienced significant drops in heart rate and blood pressure, were less agitated, slept better, needed less pain medicine, and developed a more positive outlook.

If you want to try music's healing powers for yourself, the type of music you choose should depend on the effect you want to achieve. Your heartbeat usually synchronizes itself to the rhythm of the music you're listening to.

To promote healing in the body, choose music that has an easy, flowing melody and a rhythm of 72 beats per minute or less. This rhythm is similar to the resting heart rate. Mozart's music seems to be especially beneficial because much of it, especially his slow pieces, has a relaxing effect on most people. It soothes and inspires without overexciting the body. However, if you simply can't stand Mozart, listening to him probably won't help you. The best healing effects seem to come from listening to music you enjoy.

For more serious health problems, consider consulting a music therapist. They treat a variety of health conditions. To find a qualified music therapist in your area or for more in-depth information about music therapy, contact the National Association for Music Therapy at 301-589-3300.

Get the facts so you'll feel better faster

It's especially important to know exactly how to take your medicine and when you can resume your normal activities. These two things can have a huge impact on your health. However, a recent study suggests only 57 percent of people discharged from the hospital were aware of their medicine's possible side effects. Only 58 percent knew when they could resume their normal activities.

While it is your doctor's responsibility to give you this information, it's up to you to prompt him for it if he forgets. It's also important that you make sure you understand his directions. This study also revealed that doctors think their patients understand a lot more than they actually do. That's why it's so important to ask questions. Before you leave the hospital, repeat back to him what you thought you heard him say. This is a good way to make sure there have been no misunderstandings. If you don't feel like asking questions yourself, ask a family member or trusted friend to do it for you.

In summary

The serious decision of surgery requires careful thought and planning. To make sure all goes well for you, follow the simple, seven-step plan to success:

1. Ask if there are different ways of doing the surgery you're scheduled for.

2. Find out where you'll have surgery.

3. Get your doctor to completely and clearly explain your surgery.

4. Tell your doctor about any medicines you take regularly, including aspirin.

5. Don't eat or drink anything after midnight the night before your surgery.

6. Arrange for a responsible adult to take you home afterward.

7. Dress for comfort.

For the best possible outcome, it's also important that you prepare your body for surgery. Remember Dr. Nickel's easy-to-follow plan:

- Exercise

- Eat a well-balanced diet

- Rest

- Take a multivitamin

In order to make your surgery as painless as possible, your doctor will use some sort of anesthesia. The type will depend on what kind of surgery you're having. Your doctor will be able to tell you whether your operation calls for local, regional, or general anesthesia.

Local anesthesia only numbs a specific part of your body for a short period of time. Regional anesthesia numbs a larger part of your body. With general anesthesia, which knocks you out completely, your entire body will be numb during surgery.

Before surgery, be sure you let the anesthesiologist know what medicines you're taking as well as if you drink or smoke regularly. All of these things may affect your anesthesia.

If it's possible that you may need a blood transfusion during surgery, try to donate some of your own blood in the weeks before your operation. This is the best way to reduce your risk of infection.

Your mental attitude is important to the success of your surgery. Keep your own thoughts positive and protect yourself from negative comments that may undermine your health. It's especially important that medical caregivers keep their comments positive during surgery. Negative ideas can seep into your unconscious and interfere with your healing process.

By keeping your pain under control after surgery, you'll get well faster and reduce your risk of complications. The following suggestions can help you manage your pain effectively:

- Ask your doctor what to expect after surgery.

- Discuss your pain control options before you go in for surgery.

- Talk about the pain management schedule you'll follow in the hospital.

- Don't be a silent sufferer.

- Relax your way to pain relief.

- Try alternative methods of pain relief, including massage, hot and cold packs, music, and positive thinking. Some research even suggests that listening to music may help your body heal faster.

With surgery behind you and your pain relief under control, all you need concern yourself with now is avoiding complications. This means following doctors' orders and not trying to do too much too soon. You can also avoid one of the most common complications of surgery — blood clots — by doing some simple, easy exercises while you recover in bed. See the easy-to-understand directions and illustrations on page 136.

Once your doctor says you're ready to be discharged from the hospital, you only have two things to do: Make sure you know how to take your medicines and when you can resume your normal activities. Keeping those two important points in mind, you're well on your way to a full recovery.

Food is an important part of a balanced diet.
Fran Lebowitz, American author and humorist

7

Prostate cancer prevention

Prehistoric man may or may not have suffered from prostate problems. Well-preserved ancient prostates are practically impossible to find. However, researchers think prehistoric man may have avoided the problem of prostate cancer — probably because his diet centered on fruits, vegetables, and grains. Also, he probably died of what they called old age, in his 20s or 30s, long before the prostate would have caused him any problems.

Today, it's a different story. Researchers know only too well how the problem of prostate cancer plagues modern man. The prostate is the most common site of cancer in men, and prostate cancer is the second-leading cause of death from cancer in men after lung cancer.

Over the years, people have blamed prostate cancer on any number of things, from too little sex to too much sex. Heavy drinking, having a vasectomy, and a long list of other things have also served as scapegoats.

Knowing risk factors gives you an edge

The best way to beat prostate cancer is to prevent it. And, believe it or not, many of the risks that determine whether or not you become a prostate statistic are within your control. Some risk factors you simply can't change. If you're born into a family with a history of prostate cancer, you're stuck with a slightly higher risk, even if you completely cut all family ties.

For example, a first-degree relative (such as a father or brother) with prostate cancer roughly doubles your risk. Two first-degree relatives with prostate cancer increases your risk by five times.

Some other risk factors include:

▶ **Age.** Basically the longer you live, the more likely you are to be diagnosed with prostate cancer. However, this doesn't make it any more likely that you will die from this disease.

▶ **African-American heritage.** The African-American's rate of prostate cancer is two to three times greater than the general population's. In fact, African-Americans have the highest risk of prostate cancer in the world.

Even though having risk factors you have no control over can be frustrating, just knowing what's a risk factor and what's not can give you more of a sense of control over your health.

Even better, there are other risk factors, like diet and exercise, you can control. And research suggests that what you do in those areas can make a big difference to your prostate's health. And fortunately, the list of risk factors you can't control is much shorter than the list of those you can.

Flawed gene may bear the blame

Because men with a family history of prostate cancer tend to be at greater risk themselves, researchers have long suspected that a defective gene may be at fault. Finally, they have the first proof that such a gene exists.

A combined group of researchers from Johns Hopkins University, the National Institutes of Health, and Umea University in Sweden have identified the location of the gene they think predisposes men to prostate cancer.

It appears to be a defect in the gene segment called HPC-1 (the hereditary prostate cancer 1-gene) that causes up to one-third of inherited cases of prostate cancer. Researchers estimate that about one in every 500 men has a defective version of this gene. This altered gene seems to be especially common among African-American men.

Researchers expect to face long hours in uncovering exactly which gene in the gene segment is responsible. Once they pinpoint a specific gene, they hope to be able to use that information to understand why and how prostate cancer develops and how to prevent and treat this common problem.

Cancer-proof your world

Because death rates differ among countries and even among regions of the United States, researchers suspect environmental factors may cause small tumors to grow into significant and potentially deadly cancers. Your environment may increase your risk one and a half times.

Environmental risk may not seem like it would be very easy to control. However, if researchers can pinpoint what in the environment is causing your problem, perhaps you can eliminate it. If that's not an option, moving to a safer place may be.

Following are some easy ways you can possibly lower your risk of prostate cancer.

▶ **Be careful of cadmium.** Workers in fields where they are regularly exposed to cadmium, such as welding, electroplating, and the manufacture of rubber, tires, or alkaline batteries, have slightly higher prostate cancer risks. Also, men who live in urban areas or work with industrial chemicals have a slightly higher risk. Cutting back on your exposure to cadmium also means putting out your cigarette and throwing away your chewing tobacco — forever.

▶ **Soak up some rays.** Early research indicates that exposure to sunlight may protect against prostate cancer by helping your body produce vitamin D. One study found that deaths from prostate cancer were highest where exposure to sunlight was lowest. Another study found that the active form of vitamin D may change the makeup of prostate cancer cells, making them less likely to spread.

Get at least a half hour of sunlight every day without using sunscreen, which can block your body's absorption of vitamin D. This is the best way to ensure you'll get plenty of vitamin D. It's difficult to get enough vitamin D from food, and supplements can be toxic if you take too much. If you do take supplements, the recommended amount is 400 to 800 International Units (IU) daily.

▶ **Exercise.** Experts think exercise may reduce your risk of prostate cancer by lowering testosterone levels, which tend to promote prostate growth. A recent study of almost 13,000 men provides support for this theory.

Researchers at the Cooper Clinic in Dallas found that men who burned more than 1,000 calories a week exercising were significantly less likely to be diagnosed with prostate cancer than men who didn't. Walking, swimming, and aerobics are all good exercise options.

▶ **Say no to unsafe sex.** Sex in itself won't increase your risk of prostate cancer, but there is some speculation among researchers that a sexually transmitted virus can. Although the evidence supporting the theory that the sexually transmitted virus (human papillomavirus type 16) can cause prostate cancer is slim, it won't hurt you to take precautions. Researchers suggest that you limit your number of sexual partners and use a latex condom during intercourse. If you always stick with the same partner, you may not need to use a condom for protection from the papillomavirus.

▶ **Don't panic if you've had a vasectomy.** So far, although there is a suggested link between vasectomy and prostate cancer, there is no positive proof. A review by the National Cancer Institute and the American Urological Association says it's unlikely that vasectomy raises prostate cancer risk. Based on all the evidence so far, experts say there is no need to reverse a vasectomy if you've already had one.

▶ **Save yourself with regular screening.** Although having your prostate checked regularly won't prevent you from getting prostate cancer, regular screenings can help you catch it while it's still easily treatable. For more on prostate cancer screening, see Chapter 8.

Where to go for inexpensive screenings

Many hospitals in most major cities provide annual prostate cancer screenings either free or at a reduced cost. To find out if a city near you offers this service, call the American Cancer Institute's national office at 1-800-ACS-2345. You can also find out which hospitals provide the screenings and when these services are offered.

The lean linger longer

Stay slim. Not only is fat in your diet bad for you, fat on your body is, too. According to the results from a Swedish study, your risk of prostate cancer increases right along with your body mass index. Men with a body mass index (BMI) greater than 29 have an 80 percent greater risk of developing prostate cancer than men with a BMI of less than 23.

To figure your own BMI, first calculate your height in inches. For example, if you're 5 feet 8 inches tall, this number would be 68 (12 x 5 = 60 and 60 + 8 = 68). Now square your height in inches. In this example, 68 squared would be 4,624 (68 x 68).

Next, divide your weight (in pounds) by your squared height. Let's say you weigh 150 pounds. You would divide 150 by 4,624, which equals .0324. Now multiply this number by 705 to find your BMI, which in this case would be 22.8.

Keep in mind that a high BMI does not always mean you're fat. It also takes into account your body's muscle mass. If you're a body builder, a professional athlete, or you simply work out a lot, your BMI may reflect your muscle mass more than it does body fat. However, a high BMI is still associated with a higher risk of prostate cancer. Even if your high BMI reflects more muscle mass than fat, make sure you have regular prostate screenings.

Be a gourmet, not a gourmand. How much you eat may be as important as what you eat when it comes to preventing cancer. The same Swedish study that provided the scoop on BMI and prostate cancer also found that heavy eaters have almost a four times greater risk of prostate cancer compared with more moderate eaters. So enjoy the many exquisite flavors of food like a gourmet would, but don't indulge in the gourmand's tendency to overeat.

Limit fat. Men with the highest fat intake have a 79 percent increased risk of advanced prostate cancer compared to those with the lowest intake. Men consuming the most saturated fat per day (over 35 grams) have a 60 percent greater risk of prostate cancer. Saturated fat is found mainly in animal products like cheese, butter, cream, whole milk, ice cream, and marbled meats. Some vegetable oils — palm oil, palm kernel oil, coconut oil, and cocoa butter — are also high in saturated fat. Other high fat foods to watch out for include salad dressings and oils.

Another possible reason to limit fat comes from some Canadian research currently in progress. Fat appears to soak up harmful chemicals from the environment, such as pesticides like DDT. Fat also likes to hold onto PCBs, chemicals used in electrical insulators, lubricants, plasticizers, cutting oils, and carbonless copy papers.

Although DDT and PCBs are now banned in North America, they are still used in other countries, and they're commonly found in soil, water, and food. (These complex chemicals take a very long time to break down so they tend to hang around for a while.)

The researchers speculate that these chemicals may either mimic the action of androgens, or they may increase the body's actual production of androgens. Extra androgens are something you really don't need since these male hormones are suspected of promoting prostate cancer growth.

Limit your fat intake to no more than 30 percent of your total calories. Try to reduce your intake of saturated fat to 10 percent of your total calories or less.

This means you can eat:
57 grams for a 1,700 calorie diet.
67 grams for a 2,000 calorie diet.
73 grams for a 2,200 calorie diet.
83 grams for a 2,500 calorie diet.

Trying to limit fat to 25 percent or less of your diet is a difficult goal to achieve, and it may not even be good for your health. In fact, the most recent studies suggest that it may have more negative effects on your health than keeping fat levels at 26 to 30 percent.

Fake fats hinder more than help

One of the newest fake fats on the market, olestra, marketed as Olean by Procter & Gamble, may hinder more than help your fight against prostate cancer.

Procter & Gamble openly admits that olestra interferes with your body's absorption of the fat-soluble vitamins A, D, E, and K. This may present a problem in your quest against cancer since vitamins A and E are powerful antioxidants that help protect your body from cancer.

In addition, olestra may interfere with your body's absorption of carotenoids, nutrients researchers suspect also have potent cancer-fighting abilities. One such carotenoid, lycopene, has already been associated with a reduced risk of prostate cancer in a Harvard study.

Eating as few as three small snacks containing olestra per week could drop your carotenoid levels by at least 10 percent.

In fact, epidemiologist Meir J. Stampfer of the Harvard School of Public Health estimates that eating olestra products may mean another 2,400 to 9,800 cases of prostate cancer each year.

Follow the golden rule of nutrition

To control your chances of getting prostate cancer, remember the golden rule of nutrition: Fat promotes cancer; fiber prevents it.

Protect your prostate with pizza

If you think pizza can't be a health food, think again. Pizza was among three tomato-based foods (along with tomatoes and tomato sauce) in a Harvard study that was associated with a reduced risk of prostate cancer. Tomato sauce was associated with the greatest protective benefit.

Researchers found that the risk of prostate cancer was reduced by 45 percent among men who ate at least 10 servings of tomato-based products a week. This reduction was attributed to lycopene, the substance in tomatoes that gives them their red color.

Generally, the lycopene from cooked tomato products, such as tomato paste or tomato sauce, is much more easily absorbed than from fresh tomatoes. Researchers believe that chopping and cooking tomatoes helps break down cell walls and makes the lycopene much easier to absorb.

Easy-to-make main dishes that can add lots of lycopene to your life include chili con carne, pizza, and spaghetti with tomato sauce or a tomato-based meat sauce. Ketchup can also be a good source of lycopene if you eat it fairly often. If you simply can't stand tomato-based foods, other sources of lycopene include watermelon, pink grapefruit, guava, papaya, apricots, and rose hips.

To help your body make the most use of lycopene, be sure you're getting enough zinc. A multivitamin that contains 15 milligrams (mg), the recommended dietary allowance (RDA) for zinc, should be sufficient.

Genetically engineering the perfect tomato

Gardeners have been trying to grow what they consider the perfect tomato for years: big, round, juicy, richly colored, and tasty. Scientists, however, have been working on their own version of the perfect tomato — full of disease-fighting carotenoids.

Scientists in Europe have created a tomato that has twice as much lycopene and four times as much beta carotene as an ordinary tomato. They did this by inserting a gene that helps the plant produce the carotenoids. According to researchers, the genetically altered tomatoes taste the same as any other tomato, but they may be a bit more colorful.

Since lycopene and beta carotene have both been shown in scientific studies to help prevent disease, increasing their content in foods could help people get more protection from cancer and heart disease while eating less. Scientists in other parts of the world are working on similar projects involving peppers.

While it may be some time before genetically altered foods appear in your grocery store, this scientific approach to agriculture may someday help make people a little healthier.

Fight back with food

One of the best ways to reduce your risk of prostate cancer is to eat healthy foods. That doesn't mean depriving yourself of your favorite foods. It just means including plenty of fresh fruits and vegetables in your diet and limiting fats and sugars.

If you have a lot of bad habits you think may be harming your health, work on changing them gradually rather than all at once. One easy way to start is to keep your eye on the labels of the foods you eat. This is a good way to compare different foods as far as fat, sugar, vitamin, and mineral content. Looking for lower levels of fats and sugars and higher levels of vitamins, minerals, and fiber will help you make wiser food choices.

Here are some other suggestions that can help keep your prostate and your health in tiptop shape:

Feast on fiber. Enjoy whole-grain pasta and breads and at least five servings of fruits and vegetables every day. A study of 14,000 Seventh-Day Adventist men revealed that beans, lentils, peas, tomatoes, raisins, dates, and other dried foods also appear to lower prostate cancer risk. Researchers think fiber may help reduce exposure to male hormones that tend to promote prostate growth.

Savor seafood, lean meats, and rich grain products. This will ensure that you are getting enough selenium, a powerful anti-cancer mineral. Good natural sources of selenium include bran, Brazil nuts, brewer's yeast, broccoli, cabbage, celery, chicken, cucumbers, eggs, garlic, kidney, liver, milk, mushrooms, radishes, and seafood.

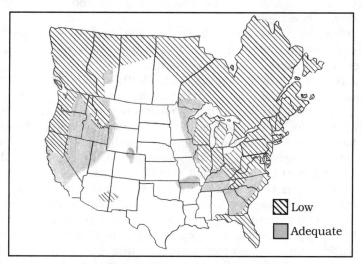

Figure 7.1. — Keep in mind that selenium levels of vegetables, grains, and nuts can vary according to where they were grown. This map shows areas of the United States and Canada where soil levels of selenium are adequate or low. Areas that aren't marked vary widely in their selenium concentration.

An easy way to boost selenium is to choose whole grains over refined foods whenever possible. Also, limit vegetable cooking time. Boiling veggies reduces their selenium content by almost half. A high-sugar diet also contributes to selenium deficiency.

Don't forget your antioxidants. Vitamins A, C, and beta carotene (which is converted to vitamin A in the body) are all-important antioxidant sources. Antioxidants sweep up unstable oxygen molecules, called free radicals, that promote cancer. Antioxidants can be harmful if taken in very high doses, so get them by eating a variety of fresh foods.

Good sources of vitamin A are deep-green and yellow vegetables and fruits, including winter squash, apricots, peaches, cantaloupe, and broccoli. There's another good reason to eat broccoli, Brussels sprouts, and other members of this plant family. A study found that these veggies may actually deactivate certain genes that could promote prostate cancer.

Good sources of vitamin C include cabbage, cauliflower, citrus fruits such as oranges and grapefruit, berries, and melon.

Sources rich in both vitamins A and C are Brussels sprouts, leafy greens, spinach, tomatoes, sweet green and red peppers, and sweet potatoes.

Other green-yellow vegetables that appear to be protective against prostate cancer include pumpkin, carrots, spinach, green leaf lettuce, and green asparagus.

Eat up vitamin E. Besides being another potent antioxidant, vitamin E may offer a little extra protection against prostate cancer. Two recent studies of male smokers who took 50 mg of vitamin E daily, compared with smokers who didn't, provide the first evidence that vitamin E might offer powerful protection against prostate cancer. Whole-grain cereals and dark-green vegetables contain vitamin E, as do wheat germ and nuts.

Tempt your taste buds with sweet strawberries. Although all fruits and vegetables are good for you, strawberries seem to offer especially strong protection against prostate cancer.

Pump up prostate protection with protease inhibitors. Protease inhibitors protect your prostate by decreasing the amount of available protein your body can digest. This is helpful because experts think excess protein may raise your cancer risk. Protease inhibitors also work like antioxidants by sweeping up free radicals that could lead to cancer.

Protease inhibitors are commonly found in seeds, rice, beans, corn, soybeans, kidney beans, chickpeas, and whole grains.

Go for some glutathione. This amino acid manufactured by your body has a remarkable ability to neutralize toxic substances before they can harm you. This role makes glutathione an effective cancer preventive. It binds with cancer-causing substances and makes them harmless.

Although your body produces glutathione, you can also get it from your diet. Fresh fruits and vegetables are the richest sources of glutathione, especially cooked asparagus, raw avocados, and cantaloupes. However, if you eat a lot of canned and processed foods, which can deplete your level of glutathione, you may want to consider a supplement.

One of the best ways to boost your level of glutathione is to take glutamine supplements. Glutamine is the most abundant amino acid in the human body. Interestingly, when taken as a supplement, glutamine is converted into glutathione in your body. This seems to work better than taking glutathione directly.

Soy saves the day

Asians typically eat a soy-saturated diet. Interestingly enough, as compared to Westerners, they also traditionally have a much lower risk of death from hormone-related cancers such as prostate cancer. However, Japanese men still develop about the same number of small prostate cancers. The only difference is Japanese men are much less likely to die from prostate cancer than Western men.

Researchers have traced soy's protective effects to phytoestrogens, plant compounds that act like or interact with estrogen hormones in animals. The two protective phytoestrogens in soy are genistein and daidzein. In addition to offering a protective benefit, animal studies suggest phytoestrogens may even be able to inhibit tumor growth. Vegetarians, who consume large amounts of phytoestrogens by way of their fruit, vegetable, and whole-grain centered diet, provide support for this theory because they too have lower rates of prostate cancer than the general population.

So, how much soy is enough? Although scientists aren't able to agree on the exact amount, they think one serving a day should offer you some protection against cancer.

Here are the average amounts of isoflavones, the estrogen-like, cancer-fighting plant substances unique to soybeans, typical servings of soy provide:

1/2 cup of soy flour = 50 mg isoflavones

1 cup of soy milk, 1 ounce of soy nuts, or 1/2 cup of tofu or tempeh = 40 mg isoflavones

1/2 cup cooked soybeans or textured vegetable protein = 35 mg isoflavones

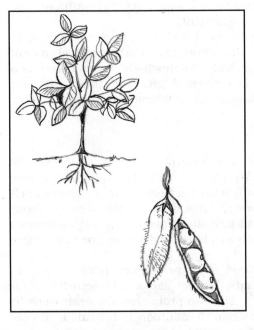

Figure 7.2 - Soybeans are known as the "greater bean" in the Chinese language.

Foods to steer clear of

While you're busy loading up on prostate-healthy foods, go easy on these:

▶ **Red meat.** Men who ate the most red meat were two and a half times more likely to develop advanced tumors. In fact, you may want to consider limiting all meat. Researchers at

Harvard Medical School found that men who ate meat five times a week were two to three times more likely to develop prostate cancer than men who only ate meat once a week.

▶ **Alcohol.** Drink alcohol in moderation if you drink it at all. Prostate cancer risk is significantly higher for men who drink 22 to 56 drinks or more per week.

▶ **Salt-cured, pickled, and smoked foods.** Limit these foods and cut back on charcoal grilling and smoking foods, which produce chemicals similar to those in cigarette smoke. The charcoal-grilled and smoked foods absorb these chemicals.

Good news about green tea

For prostate protection, think green — green tea, that is.

Previously, both animal and human studies provided convincing evidence that green tea can inhibit a wide variety of cancers, including stomach, esophageal, gastrointestinal, liver, lung, and pancreatic. The latest in a long line of studies suggests that the goodness of green tea may also help prevent prostate cancer.

In a lab test at Case Western Reserve University in Cleveland, researchers found that a powerful antioxidant in green tea called epigallocatechin-3-gallate killed prostate cancer cells in both mice and humans yet left healthy cells unharmed.

According to lead researcher Dr. Hasan Mukhtar, one cup of green tea contains about 100 to 200 mg of this anti-tumor antioxidant. How much is enough to possibly offer cancer protection? About four cups a day, estimates Dr. Mukhtar.

The next time you turn to tea for a quick afternoon pick-me-up, go for the green to keep your golden glow of health.

Antioxidants combat cancer

New research suggests that free radicals may be the villain in yet another disease — prostate cancer.

But that's not the only twist to this radical theory. Researchers think female hormones may also be at fault. Traditionally, male sex hormones, such as testosterone, have been blamed for encouraging the development of prostate cancer.

Although male hormones, called androgens, must be present for prostate cancer to develop, researchers think estrogen may also play a role. If male hormones, such as testosterone, were primarily responsible for prostate cancer, it appears that young men at the peak of their testosterone production would be the most likely to develop prostate cancer. However, this is not the case. Prostate cancer tends to strike mostly older men.

Interestingly enough, it's in older men that estrogen levels begin to rise while testosterone levels fall, which leads some researchers to conclude that estrogen may play a part in the development of prostate cancer. Researchers suggest it may be the subtle shift in estrogen that leads to the development of prostate cancer. In fact, animal studies show that giving male animals both estrogen and testosterone at the same time tends to promote prostate cancer development.

Researchers speculate that it's the breakdown of estrogen that unleashes the free radicals that damage DNA and ultimately lead to cancer.

The good news is that a healthy antioxidant diet may help prevent this problem. Antioxidants sweep up those free radicals.

Vitamin E, lycopene, and selenium, all well-known antioxidants, show great promise for heading off prostate cancer. Researchers believe antioxidants like these may be able to slow down prostate cancer's progress or even prevent it.

Genistein, a compound in soy foods, may help protect against prostate cancer by acting as an anti-estrogen.

Possible key to prostate cancer prevention

Researchers think they may have found the key to prostate cancer prevention — all wrapped up in a little package of protein.

A new study shows that one out of four men has high levels of a growth protein called IGF-1 (insulin-like growth factor-1), which has been linked to a greater risk of prostate cancer. Men with the highest IGF-1 levels were over four times more likely to be diagnosed with prostate cancer than men with the lowest levels.

Early evidence also suggests the protein may encourage prostate tumors to be more aggressive. This may explain why

More praise for finasteride

In addition to relieving the irritating symptoms of BPH, as well as being the newest cure on the block for baldness, researchers think finasteride (the brand name is Proscar), a drug commonly used to treat men with enlarged prostates) may also help prevent prostate cancer.

Right now, the Prostate Cancer Clinical Trial (PCCT) is underway to test this theory. Researchers are studying 18,000 men age 55 and older to see if Proscar can indeed prevent prostate cancer.

One-half of the men are taking 5 mg of finasteride a day. The other half are taking a placebo (a fake pill). After the seven-year trial is completed, the prostate cancer rates of the two groups will be compared.

Researchers think finasteride will prevent prostate cancer much the same way it relieves the symptoms of an enlarged prostate — by reducing levels of the hormone dihydrotestosterone (DHT), which promotes the development of prostate cancer.

African-American men die of prostate cancer more often than white men. Generally, African-Americans have higher IGF-1 levels.

IGF-1 may also explain why overweight men appear to be more at risk of prostate cancer than normal weight men. Generally, overeaters have higher IGF-1 levels, too.

Currently, researchers are conducting animal studies to determine if drugs that lower the level of the protein may actually prevent prostate cancer. One day, researchers may also be able to use the protein to predict which men will develop prostate cancer.

Even though this research is in its infant stages, it appears to have important implications for men right now, especially men who take the anti-aging growth hormones that have been widely promoted lately. The growth hormone raises IGF-1 levels, which researchers think may translate into a higher risk of prostate cancer. The bottom line: To protect yourself from prostate cancer, don't take growth hormones. A wrinkle or two is well worth a few more good years.

In summary

Although you can't control all your risk factors for prostate cancer, you can control more of them than you might think. While things like age and family history are totally out of your hands, you can take charge of several things that may contribute to prostate cancer risk.

First, watch out for cadmium, a metal used in welding, electroplating, and in making alkaline batteries. Cutting out cadmium also means tossing your cigarettes and your chewing tobacco.

Be sure to sprinkle lots of sunshine into your life, a little every day if possible. This helps your body produce vitamin D, which is important in helping your body defend itself against prostate cancer.

While you're out enjoying the sunshine, squeeze in a little exercise, too. Studies show that men who use more than 1,000 calories a week exercising have lower risks of prostate cancer.

Finally, be sure your sex is safe and don't neglect your regular prostate screening. Generally, the earlier a cancer is found, the easier it is to treat.

After you've cleaned up the cancer risks in your environment, get to work on your diet. Following a few simple diet dos and don'ts may offer you significant prostate protection. The bottom line: Limit fat and calories. While there's no need to starve, stuffing yourself won't help you stay slim (another way of lowering prostate cancer risk). And forget trying to fool your body by eating fake fats, such as olestra. Your body doesn't believe for a minute that the stuff is real food. Also, eating several snacks a week that contain olestra may actually raise your prostate cancer risk by interfering with absorption of several important vitamins.

Other prostate protectors include lycopene, zinc, fiber, selenium, vitamin A, vitamin C, vitamin E, soy, and green tea.

While you're loading up on prostate-healthy foods, like wholegrains, lean meat, seafood, and fresh fruits and vegetables, here are some items you'll want to limit: red meat; alcohol; and salt-cured, pickled, and smoked foods.

Although cleaning up your environment and eating prostate-healthy foods are no guarantee you'll avoid prostate cancer, they can at least give you a good head start. Throw in a positive attitude and you're all set to make the most of your life today and every day.

*I find there's a lot of fear,
not only about the ravages of the disease
but also about the rectal exam.
But these tests can save your life.*
Bob Watson, prostate cancer survivor
and general manager of the New York Yankees

8

Screening for prostate cancer

To test or not to test

Although doctors generally have their individual opinions about prostate cancer screening (testing men with no symptoms for the presence of cancer), most will present the facts to you and let you make the final choice. If they feel strongly about your situation for some reason or another (if you have a family history of prostate cancer, for example) they may strongly encourage screening. If you have no apparent risk factors and no suspicious prostate problems, they may strongly discourage you.

However, the final choice is up to you. To make the decision that's best for your health and that's most comfortable for you, it's important to consider these issues before you're faced with making a choice.

How to decide what's right for you

As with most cancers, prostate cancer is easier to cure in the early stages. If it is allowed to spread, your chances of survival plummet. Your doctor can give you a digital rectal exam (DRE), and if you have a tumor, he may be able to feel it. He may also give you a prostate specific antigen (PSA) test. PSA is a protein that is secreted into your prostatic ducts during ejaculation. Normally, very little PSA enters your bloodstream. If you have an abnormality in your prostate, like a tumor, more of the protein may escape into your bloodstream.

According to some researchers, if every man follows the recommendation of the American Cancer Society by getting an annual screening starting at age 50, the proportion of localized or potentially curable cancers can be increased from about 40 percent without screening to more than 95 percent.

Despite statistics that suggest a definite benefit of prostate cancer screening, plenty of other statistics do not. In fact, no studies so far have conclusively demonstrated that screening with the DRE and PSA test actually lowers the risk of death from prostate cancer. In addition, some researchers warn that screening and treatment may lead to a poorer quality of life due to side effects of surgery, such as incontinence and impotence, rather than a longer life.

Still, at this time, the only way doctors know how to reduce death from prostate cancer is by screening and early diagnosis.

Before you have the screening tests, you need to decide if you'd be willing to undergo treatment if cancer is found. Possible side effects of treatment for prostate cancer include incontinence and impotence. More than 25 percent of the men treated with surgery or chemotherapy develop impotence. About 10 percent or more become incontinent.

A couple of other considerations to keep in mind: If you're over age 75 or your life expectancy is less than 10 years, chances are you may not benefit that much from these tests. While the tests may find cancer, you may discover that the compromises you have to make in terms of quality of life are not worth a few extra years. Plus, the cancers may be insignificant, so you may end up making sacrifices for a cancer that wasn't going to kill you anyway.

Medicare must pay

Starting in the year 2000, Medicare must pay for prostate screening tests for all men age 50 and older.

Get the facts — set your mind at ease

Once you welcome your 50th birthday, your doctor is likely to start recommending that you have a yearly DRE along with a PSA test.

The American Cancer Society and the American Urological Association recommend annual PSA and DRE tests for all men over 50. If you are African-American or have a family history of prostate cancer, these associations recommend you begin testing at age 40.

For most men, the prospect of a prostate exam is not a pleasant thought. Although it's easy to imagine all sorts of horrors, most men find the experience not nearly as bad as they thought it would be. Since most men say they don't dread the exams as much if they know exactly what to expect, this chapter can help ease your mind.

If you have any other worries, don't hesitate to bring them up with your doctor. All good doctors are more than willing to take the time to calm your fears and explain the procedures clearly.

Put your health to the test

At the beginning of your exam, you'll usually have to answer a few questions about your general health. (You can find more

---

Prostate exams: Early detection saves lives

Chances are, if you're a man, by the time you're 80 years old, you will develop the beginnings of prostate cancer. Prostate cancer develops in 40 percent of men over age 50 and up to 70 percent of men over 80.

While prostate cancer is fairly prevalent, the good news is you don't have to die from it. You can catch it early with the proper tests. Plus, a low-fat, high-fiber diet reduces the risk that microscopic prostate cancers will spread and become life-threatening.

Symptoms of prostate cancer often don't appear until it is so far advanced that treatment can't stop it. Many men choose to test despite the ongoing controversy. They know the sooner cancer is found, the sooner it can be stopped and the greater their chances of survival.

information on these questions in Chapter 2). Once that's over, your doctor will want to do a general physical check. He'll poke and prod your stomach and pelvic areas to check for swollen or tender spots.

If you've decided that a DRE and a PSA test are the route you want to take, you're now ready to move into those portions of the exam.

Why you don't need to fear the DRE

You may find it reassuring to know that the digital rectal exam is hardly ever associated with agonizing pain. (If it is, that's a pretty good sign you have a prostate infection.)

In addition, many men fear that the exam will cause an embarrassing erection. Although that rarely occurs, you can bet you won't be the first or the last to have that experience. Considering the consequences of not having the exam, most men find a little embarrassment much easier to live with than a condition that interferes with their enjoyment of life or that threatens their very existence.

For any suspected prostate problem or as part of your yearly checkup, the rectal exam is a regular part of the routine. Although this exam is uncomfortable, it causes more discomfort than actual pain. (Doctors who have had the exam themselves vouch for this.) As much as you may hate the idea of this exam, some experts swear by it, saying it's your best defense against prostate cancer.

To check your prostate, the doctor will ask you to undress and bend over. Some doctors may have you lie on your side on the examining table. He will then insert a gloved, lubricated finger about 4 inches into your rectum and press down.

During the rectal exam, your doctor will try to determine if your prostate has any hard lumps, which may suggest cancer, or if any areas feel tender and soft, which may indicate infection. A healthy prostate feels firm and elastic to the touch.

If your doctor suspects an infection, he will probably want to do a urine test. For the most accurate diagnosis, most doctors use the segmented urine culture. (For a full description, see Chapter 14, *Diagnostic tests*.) If your doctor feels a hard or firm area, he'll probably suggest a biopsy.

How the PSA test spots prostate cancer

The main purpose of prostate specific antigen (PSA) is to liq-uefy semen after ejaculation so sperm may be released on their journey to find an available egg to fertilize. In the 1980s, researchers discovered that PSA was useful for determining if treatment for prostate cancer had removed all malignant tissue. They also used PSA to monitor for the recurrence of cancer.

However, researchers quickly realized PSA could be just as use-ful in detecting early cancer as in monitoring its recurrence. Since the early 1990s, doctors have used PSA to test for prostate cancer.

The PSA test measures your level of prostate specific antigen, a protein made primarily by the prostate. In all healthy men, a small amount of PSA protein passes into the bloodstream from the prostate. Larger amounts may pass through if some abnor-mality of the prostate gland, such as benign prostatic hyperplasia (BPH) or cancer, has altered the structure of the gland, allowing more PSA to get into the bloodstream. Extra PSA floating around

Easing the discomfort of the rectal exam

Dr. Raymond Roberge of Pittsburgh finds that for many men the most uncomfortable part of the rectal exam is the initial insertion of a finger into the rectum. To ease this process, he places his finger at the opening of the anus and asks the patient to cough forcefully. This causes the anus to contract and relax and results in the finger being drawn gradually into the rectum with very little discomfort. During the exam, it may also help to lessen discomfort if you strain downward as if you were having a bowel movement.

Your doctor probably already knows this technique and may use it during your exams. If he doesn't, you may want to suggest this tech-nique to your doctor the next time you're scheduled for a rectal exam. The act of coughing also tends to take your mind off that initial irri-tation.

in your bloodstream won't hurt you. High PSA levels simply signal you have a problem with your prostate.

Your doctor may use this test to confirm his suspicions of either BPH or prostate cancer. Usually, the PSA test identifies those cancers that are still confined to the prostate and are still easily treatable.

"What the PSA test does is alert the physician that a man may have something wrong with his prostate," says Max Robinowitz, M.D., medical officer in FDA's Center for Devices and Radiological Health. "The doctor must then decide if more testing is needed to identify the problem."

If cancer is present and cancer cells have left the prostate and moved to other areas of the body, your blood levels of PSA are likely to be higher. In general, the higher your PSA, the greater your risk of cancer.

Double inspection gives you double protection

A PSA test can detect the presence of a tumor as much as five years sooner than other tests, such as the digital rectal exam (DRE). Despite this, the best way to detect prostate cancer is to do the two tests together.

PSA is actually considered a method of measuring risk rather than actually detecting cancer. It cannot be considered a definite indicator of cancer. About 20 to 40 percent of patients with proven prostate cancers had normal PSA levels. The American Cancer Society recommends you have both DRE and PSA tests every year after age 50. They suggest you start testing even sooner if you are African-American or have a family history of prostate cancer. The two procedures done together in addition to ultrasound-guided biopsy can increase detection of prostate cancer by 70 percent.

Prepare properly for your PSA test

If you know ahead of time that you're going to have a PSA test, don't have sex for at least two days. Ejaculation more recent than that may skew your results, making your PSA read higher than it would normally.

Sexes battle over prostate exams

When it comes to being screened for prostate cancer, men and women have dramatically different views.

Nine out of 10 women are in favor of their husbands having annual prostate screening exams. Only three out of 10 men agree with the women. The other seven out of 10 say they'd prefer not to have a prostate screening exam. Of course, women may be more inclined to favor the screening since they aren't the ones who have to put up with the digital rectal exam once a year.

Men and women also differ when it comes to quality of life vs. quantity. Men say they prefer a shorter life over treatment side effects, such as incontinence and impotence. Women, on the other hand, just want their husbands to hang around as long as humanly possible.

Although most experts agree that having a DRE before a PSA test won't affect your results significantly, it may raise them slightly. To get the most accurate results, you may want to wait 48 to 72 hours after your rectal exam before you have the PSA test. Prostate massage and transrectal ultrasonography may also slightly affect PSA levels.

Prostate biopsy usually affects PSA levels, so you should wait at least four weeks after having a prostate biopsy before having a PSA test to make sure your doctor gets the most accurate reading.

It's also important to keep in mind that the prostate drug finasteride (used to treat BPH) can skew PSA results. Finasteride can make PSA levels look lower than they would be if you weren't taking the drug. This could mean your doctor might miss diagnosing and delaying treatment of a cancer that actually was present. If you've been taking finasteride for six to 12 months and your PSA levels haven't dropped any, you should be examined for prostate cancer.

Once you're ready for your test, your doctor or nurse will take a small sample of blood. It will go to a laboratory where they will measure the amount of PSA in your blood using a special procedure called immunoassay. Your results will be reported as nanograms per milliliter of blood, usually written as ng/mL.

Understanding PSA levels

Normal PSA levels have been typically defined as being around 4 ng/mL. If you have a PSA between 4 and 10 ng/mL, the chances that you have prostate cancer are 20 to 50 percent. If your PSA level is over 10 ng/mL, you are 50 to 75 percent more likely to have prostate cancer, and if your PSA level goes over 20 ng/mL, there is a 90 percent chance you have prostate cancer.

Although normal PSA levels fall within a fairly narrow range, there's no need to panic if yours don't. There could be any number of reasons for a raised PSA that don't indicate cancer.

For example, an enlarged prostate often produces more PSA, creating higher blood levels of the protein. This may also occur when infection damages the prostate lining and allows more than normal amounts of PSA to be released. A urinary tract disorder can also raise PSA levels.

In addition, problems that aren't really related to the prostate can affect PSA levels. For example, researchers recently noted that acute viral hepatitis (inflammation of the liver caused by a virus) can also raise PSA levels. During a young man's bout of hepatitis, his PSA levels peaked at 28 ng/mL, an amount typically assumed to be caused by cancer. If you have unexplained increases in your PSA levels, it could be a case of underlying liver disease. Low testosterone levels also appear to lower PSA levels and may even affect prostate tumors, making them undetectable during a DRE exam.

Even age and race influence PSA levels. As men age, their PSA levels tend to increase. Also, PSA levels are higher and more varied among African-American men. Based on the so-called "normal" PSA levels, over 40 percent of the cases of prostate cancer in African-American men would not be detected. Also, PSA levels are higher among African-American men with newly diagnosed prostate cancer than they are among white men.

One way to improve the accuracy of the PSA test is to use it along with a table, such as the one that follows, which shows normal PSA ranges for men according to age and race. Following these new guidelines would help older African-American men avoid unnecessary surgery while catching prostate cancer earlier in African-American men in their 40s and 50s.

If your PSA is higher than normal for your age and race, your doctor will probably suggest a transrectal ultrasound and possibly a biopsy.

PSA levels for age and race

Age (years)	Upper limit of normal serum PSA (ng/mL)		
	African-American	Asian	White
40-49	2.0	2.0	2.5
50-59	4.0	3.0	3.5
60-69	4.5	4.0	4.5
70-79	5.5	5.0	6.5

Vashi, AR, Oesterling JE, Percent free prostate-specific antigen: entering a new era in the detection of prostate cancer. Mayo Clinic Proceedings 1997; 72:337-44. Reprinted with permission.

Rate your chance of cancer

Based on the results of your DRE and PSA tests, the Prostate Health Council put together a chart that shows how likely you are to have cancer.

Digital rectal exam	PSA blood level		
	0-4 ng/mL	4-10 ng/mL	More than 10 ng/mL
Normal	Low	Medium	High
Abnormal*	Medium	High	High

*A lump or hard area in the prostate.

Prostate Health Council of the American Foundation for Urologic Disease. Reprinted with permission.

Uncovering problems in PSA testing

The problem with the PSA test as it's used today is that it isn't specific or sensitive enough to be a really good cancer detector. Among men with organ-confined prostate cancer, 43 percent have a PSA value within the normal range (0.0 to 4.0 ng/mL). Of men with BPH, 25 percent have a PSA above normal (more than 4.0 ng/mL).

Because a number of other causes, including prostatitis, can also increase PSA levels, many men undergo the unnecessary stress and physical discomfort of a biopsy to rule out cancer. Also, a significant number of men with normal PSA levels actually do have prostate cancer.

To make PSA a more reliable way of detecting prostate cancer, researchers are developing new ways of measuring PSA that they hope will more accurately reflect the presence of cancer and cut back on unnecessary testing.

Promising ways to make PSA tests more accurate

Free vs. bound PSA. PSA exists in two forms: free and bound. One way doctors can more clearly determine whether or not cancer is actually present is by comparing the amount of free PSA to total PSA.

Free and bound PSA are identified by whether or not they are attached to a protein. Free or unbound PSA is not attached to a protein; bound PSA is attached to a protein. A low percent of free PSA and a high percent of bound PSA suggest cancer.

One study found a higher likelihood of cancer when free PSA made up 20 percent or less of total PSA. If the free PSA test is approved by the FDA (and it looks as though it probably will be in the near future), it could potentially save needless anxiety and discomfort for almost 1 million men per year.

In addition, it could save the $2,000 cost of performing a biopsy if the regular PSA test is high. A recent study conducted at Washington University suggests free PSA testing may reduce unnecessary biopsies by 20 percent. This test could be especially beneficial for African-American men, whose cancers are less likely to be detected using standard PSA ranges.

PSA density. In order to effectively distinguish prostate cancer in men with small glands from BPH in men with larger prostate glands, researchers developed PSA density.

This test is most useful for distinguishing prostate cancer from BPH in men who have PSAs between 4.0 ng/mL and 10 ng/mL and a normal DRE. The PSA density may help avoid an unnecessary biopsy by distinguishing those men at high risk of prostate cancer from those men who probably have BPH.

This measurement is determined by dividing your PSA number by the volume of your prostate. An ultrasound scan will calculate your prostate volume. The higher your PSA density, the greater your risk of cancer. Research suggests that a PSA density greater than .15 points to a high risk of cancer.

One of the problems with measuring PSA density is that it's difficult to get an accurate measurement of prostate volume using ultrasound. Also, repeat examinations of the same person may show test results that vary by as much as 15 percent.

PSA velocity. Also known as serial PSA testing, the velocity measures annual changes in PSA levels. PSA levels will rise more rapidly in a man with cancer than in a man without it. This test is useful in detecting prostate cancer in men whose PSA falls below normal levels.

However, PSA velocity needs to be monitored over a one-and-a-half to two-year period before it can accurately detect the presence of prostate cancer. An increase of more than .75 ng/mL per year suggests cancer. If you fall into that category, you'll probably need a biopsy.

Resist cancer with regular screenings

Although some men may need screening every year, men with PSA levels below 2 ng/mL and a normal DRE can probably safely go two years before having another screening test. This was the conclusion of researchers who reviewed the progress of 312 men who were part of the Baltimore Longitudinal Study of Aging. However, if your initial PSA measurement was greater than 2.0 or you're considered high-risk for prostate cancer, yearly screening is still your best option.

Since about 70 percent of men between the ages of 50 and 70 years have PSA levels less than 2 ng/mL, screening every two years can save many men a lot of anxiety and aggravation. More importantly, it may also help cut down on the diagnosis of

New blood test may work better than the PSA

While the PSA test has made it possible to detect more prostate cancers than ever before, researchers still say about 40 percent of men with prostate cancer don't have elevated PSA levels. For those men, a so-called "normal" PSA test offers a false sense of security.

A new blood test that measures human glandular kallikrein may come to the rescue. Researchers at the Mayo Clinic in Rochester, Minn., have developed a blood test that identifies high concentrations of kallikrein in the bloodstream. Like PSA, kallikrein is also a protein produced by the prostate. The researchers think kallikrein may play some part in the development and progression of prostate cancer.

At this time, kallikrein is still in early testing stages. Although this is just one of many new tests being developed that researchers hope will be more accurate than the PSA exam, early results indicate that kallikrein may be at least as good as PSA at predicting prostate cancer. Researchers are hoping further tests will find that kallikrein can ferret out those cancers the PSA test fails to find.

insignificant cancers. As an added bonus, it can mean significant savings for you and your health care system.

You needn't worry about developing an uncontrollable cancer during that time either. If you have PSA levels that are 2 ng/mL or less, you have less than a 4 percent chance that your PSA levels will rise to between 4.0 ng/mL and 5.0 ng/mL. If you develop cancer and your PSA levels rise to that range, your cancer will still be curable about 90 percent of the time.

If you're African-American, however, these study results may not apply to you since the majority of the men in this study were white. Also, you may want to go with yearly screenings since African-Americans are generally at higher risk of prostate cancer.

Other tests you may need to take

Once a DRE or PSA test suggests the presence of cancer, doctors like to do a few more tests to confirm their suspicions.

Transrectal ultrasonography (TRUS). Your urologist will use TRUS to determine the size of your prostate and identify areas that may be cancerous. If your doctor decides a biopsy is needed, he will use TRUS to help him guide the biopsy needle.

During TRUS, you will lie on your side while a probe is inserted about 3 to 4 inches up into your rectum. The probe makes images of your prostate and surrounding tissues as it is being removed from the rectum.

This procedure is usually done on an outpatient basis and only takes about 15 to 20 minutes. Most of the time, anesthesia is not required.

Biopsy. If your DRE revealed an area of hardness in your prostate or your PSA was over 10 ng/mL, your doctor will probably want to do a biopsy. This involves inserting a small needle through the rectum and up into the prostate. Your urologist will usually take four to six samples of tissue. A pathologist (a doctor who specializes in diagnosing abnormal changes in tissue samples) will examine this tissue and look for cancer cells.

With the development of the spring-loaded biopsy gun, biopsies are much less painful than in the past. Also, ultrasound allows the needle to be positioned more precisely, which also means less discomfort.

Recently, researchers also discovered that an injection of lidocaine, a local anesthetic, near the nerves that supply the prostate can significantly lessen pain during a biopsy. Using lidocaine may also mean your doctor can get more accurate biopsies since you won't move around as much during the procedure. However, many doctors don't regularly use lidocaine since the injection can be more painful than the biopsy itself.

Normally, you will receive antibiotics both before and after your biopsy to prevent infection. Besides infection, other temporary complications may include a little rectal bleeding and blood in the semen. You should receive your biopsy results within three to five days.

As accurate as biopsy results can be, they are never 100 percent guaranteed. The difficulty in detecting prostate cancer cells is that they tend to spread out instead of forming a mass or hard lump, like other cancers, that's easier to find. What this means is that even if your biopsy comes back negative, meaning no cancer was found, your doctor may want you to have another biopsy if your DRE was very suggestive of cancer or if your PSA was over 10 ng/mL.

What makes detection even more difficult is that biopsies don't always come back strongly negative or strongly positive. Sometimes, they come back rather wishy-washy. Technically, this wishy-washy response is referred to as prostatic intra-epithelial neoplasia (PIN). This response shows tissue that doesn't look like cancer, but it doesn't look exactly harmless (benign) either. In fact, PIN are abnormal cells that have a strong link to cancer. If your biopsy points out PIN, you may need another biopsy. That's because about half the time another biopsy will find cancer.

Bogus biopsy scare

The possibility that you may have prostate cancer is scary enough. What's worse is that you've heard reports that biopsies can actually cause cancer.

The truth is biopsies don't cause cancer. However, if cancer is present in your prostate, a biopsy may spread it to other tissue. Now for the good news: This was a rare problem in the past and it's practically nonexistent today. In fact, you're almost guaranteed it won't happen unless your doctor uses an outdated technique to obtain a prostate biopsy sample.

In the past, doctors often inserted a needle through the perineum (the area between the scrotum and anus) up into the prostate to retrieve a sample of prostate tissue. The problem occurred when cancer was present in the prostate and part of the sample escaped from the needle on the way out, resulting in "seeding" the perineal tissues with cancer cells. Cancer contained in the prostate is much easier to treat than cancer outside the prostate, so letting it escape into other tissues is dangerous.

However, because doctors today typically use the transrectal approach to obtain a sample of prostate tissue, cancer cells do not have a chance to escape into surrounding tissue and spread the cancer. If you're concerned about the possibility that a biopsy could spread cancer, discuss your fears with your doctor and ask him if he uses the transrectal approach. If he doesn't, find a doctor who does.

Whatever you do, don't let the fear that a biopsy may spread cancer stop you from getting a biopsy your doctor says you need. In cases of prostate cancer, a biopsy is essential for your doctor to properly diagnose and classify your cancer and give you the treatment you need. Not getting timely treatment is much more dangerous to your health than the slighter than slight possibility that a prostate biopsy may spread cancer.

A question of survival: Does screening help?

Does prostate cancer screening have any effect on long-term survival?

Part of the controversy over screening comes because no one really knows the answer to this question. However, two studies are currently in progress that hope to shed some light on this issue.

Sponsored by the National Cancer Institute, the Prostate, Lung, Colorectal, and Ovarian Cancer Screening Trial (PLCO) hopes to prove decisively that screening either does or does not affect life span. This large-scale study of 148,000 men and women ages 55 through 74 from 10 different areas across the United States will provide screening tests for half the participants. The other half will just receive their regular medical care. Results from this study should be available within the next 11 years.

Until then, you will have to make your own decision about whether the potential life-extending possibilities of the DRE and PSA exams are worth the risks of prostate cancer treatment.

Know your next step

If your screening tests suggest you have a prostate in perfect health, go home. No use standing around the doctor's office waiting until they do find something wrong with you.

If, on the other hand, your tests point to prostate cancer, don't panic. Prostate cancer is not necessarily a death sentence, but it does mean you're going to have to take a good look at your health and your priorities. You've got some decisions to make. For a guide to get you through the maze of information you're going to encounter, turn to Chapter 9.

In summary

To be screened or not screened for prostate cancer is a very confusing question. With doctors so divided over the issue, it doesn't make it any easier to decide. However, unless you are clearly at risk for prostate cancer, such as African-American men and men with a family history of prostate cancer, this is one choice you're going to have to make for yourself. While your doctor can offer guidance, even he has no clear answers — because no clear answers yet exist.

Basically, the screening issue boils down to a couple of pros and cons.

Pros

- Screening does find small cancers.

- Cancer is more easily cured in the early stages.

- Most of the cancers found by the DRE and PSA exam become deadly after a period of 10 to 15 years.

Cons

- There isn't enough data available to prove that prostate cancer screening saves a significant number of lives. Because prostate cancer is slow growing, it will probably take many years to see what effect the screening tests really have. Researchers do not expect this information to be available until after the turn of the century.

- Most cancerous prostate growths do not cause death. Although one-third of men over 50 have some form of prostate cancer, only 6 to 10 percent of these men have the deadly type. Only 3 percent of men die of it. The problem with detection tests today is that they cannot accurately detect which cancers will be deadly and which won't.

- The stress and anxiety of screening puts quite a strain on some men.

- The side effects of treatment for prostate cancer can be severe. Some men find the incontinence or impotence they experience decreases their quality of life too much to be worth a few extra years.

If you decide in favor of screening, your first step will be the digital rectal exam (DRE). Your doctor will feel your prostate to determine if you have any hard lumps that could indicate cancer.

Your next step will be a blood test that measures the levels of prostate specific antigen (PSA) in your body. PSA is a protein produced primarily by the prostate. Levels higher than 4 ng/mL suggest a possible prostate problem. This could be cancer or it could be a case of BPH, a common benign condition of the prostate discussed in Chapters 4 and 5. Other health problems, such as hepatitis, can also affect PSA levels.

If either your DRE or your PSA is abnormal, your doctor will probably want to do a transrectal ultrasound (TRUS) and biopsy to confirm if cancer is present.

If a diagnosis of cancer is made, your doctor will want to do further tests that will help him determine the stage of your cancer. Your cancer stage will help your doctor decide which treatment options will be best for you. Turn to Chapter 9 for more information on cancer stages and treatment options.

*I had never really heard of this disease ...
How many other men were out there who didn't know
to go to their doctor and get checked?*
Former Senator Bob Dole
on his prostate cancer diagnosis in 1991

The first thing you do is learn about the enemy.
General H. Norman Schwarzkopff, Gulf War hero,
talking about his prostate cancer diagnosis

9

Diagnosis cancer

It's official. Your doctor says he's found cancer in your prostate. The shock of the diagnosis seems overwhelming. You expected symptoms — some sign.

Unfortunately, prostate cancer is not often signaled by symptoms. Early stages of prostate cancer usually cause no readily apparent problems. In later stages, symptoms may mimic those of BPH — except that they appear more abruptly. As cancer enlarges the prostate, you may experience urinary frequency, hesitancy, urgency, and a need to get up several times during the night to urinate.

A decrease in the firmness of your erections or total impotence suggests prostate cancer may have spread to the nerves that control the erection process. Severe back pain may mean the cancer has spread to the bones of your vertebrae. You may also have pain in your pelvis or upper thighs, blood in the urine, and painful urination. Bone pain is a sign of progressive prostate cancer.

Although a diagnosis of cancer is frightening, it's far from being a death sentence. However, many people seem to die from fear of cancer rather than the cancer itself. Although denial and resignation are common reactions to a diagnosis of cancer, you need to move beyond those emotions to wage an effective battle against this disease. Becoming informed is the first step in your fight against prostate cancer.

10 crucial questions to ask your doctor about cancer

The first step to gaining control over your cancer is understanding it. These 10 questions can give you a clearer idea of where you stand with your cancer. It may help if you write the answers down and keep them somewhere so you can access them easily. Although these won't be the only questions you'll want to ask your doctor, they can give you the basic information you need to begin fighting back against prostate cancer.

- How did you diagnose my cancer?

- What is the stage and grade of my cancer?

- How likely is it that the cancer has spread beyond my prostate? Where has the cancer spread? What are my chances of a cure?

- What are my chances of surviving?

- What other tests do you recommend? Why?

- What are my treatment choices? Which do you recommend and why?

- What side effects and complications can I expect from treatment?

- Which treatments are most and least likely to cause impotence and incontinence?

- If my cancer is cured, what are the chances that it will recur?

- Do I need to follow a special diet before, during, or after my cancer treatment?

Because no one takes your health to heart the way you do, it's important to take the time to get your questions answered to your satisfaction. The answers may hold the key to your cure.

The bad news and the good news
about prostate cancer

Prostate cancer is an equal opportunity tumor. From you or your neighbor down the street to comedian Jerry Lewis and actor Sidney Poitier, it affects about 300,000 men a year. It's also an equal opportunity killer, taking the lives of about 45,000 men a year — both the famous and the not-so-famous.

Although researchers haven't definitely decided on a particular prostate cancer trigger, the cancer occurs when prostate cancer cells start multiplying uncontrollably. In BPH, cells also multiply rapidly, eventually to the point that their sheer number puts a real squeeze on the urethra.

However, cancer differs from benign (generally harmless) cell growth (such as BPH) in two important ways. Cancer eventually spreads beyond its organ of origin, and it is ultimately a destructive disease, destroying the very tissue that supports it.

Besides destroying its organ of origin, it eventually spreads into other tissues and organs and destroys them as well. Also, cells from the original cancer may spread via the body's blood and lymph systems to other areas where it forms new satellite tumors that grow independently.

A normal cell becomes cancerous in two steps. First, the cell is damaged and its basic genetic instructions are altered. Second, something occurs that activates the damaged (cancerous) cells. This may occur days or decades after the cell is damaged. Activators can include a variety of things, from too much dietary fat to certain chemicals.

Once a cell becomes cancerous, it passes its malignant characteristics on to all its offspring cells. Soon you have a small group of abnormal cells. These cells multiply much more rapidly than the surrounding cells and they refuse to perform the designated task of all their other host tissue's cells. Basically, cancer cells toss off their former duties and become parasites. They contribute nothing to help their host organ function, but they continue to consume nutrients.

There is some good news about prostate cancer. Uncommon in men under the age of 50, prostate cancer is generally slow growing. This means if you catch the cancer early enough and treat it aggressively, you have a very good chance of being cured.

Get the facts to make the right decisions

All the questions running through your mind return to a familiar refrain, "What do I do now?" At first the answer may seem clear. Get that cancer out and get it out now!

Although fear may steer you to that choice, it may not be your best option. The first thing you want to do — especially before you panic and make rash decisions you may regret later — is to classify your cancer. That means figuring out the grade and stage of your cancer. This tells you where the cancer is and how likely it is to spread. These facts can help you make better decisions about how you want to treat your cancer.

A number of tests can help determine where your cancer is. See Chapter 14 for a complete discussion of these tests.

Make the most of a second opinion

After a diagnosis of cancer, it's essential that you seek a second opinion. This doesn't mean the first doctor's diagnosis was incorrect or his suggested treatment was inappropriate, although that can happen.

However, you're making a decision that may mean the difference between life and death, so you need to be sure you've explored all possible options. You also need to be sure you've found the medical team that will best meet your needs. This means seeking at least a second, and possibly a third or fourth, opinion.

Three quick tips will help you make the most of additional opinions that you seek.

First, make sure you're seeing a board-certified urologist or radiotherapist who specializes in oncology. These doctors regularly deal with prostate cancer so they're most likely to be up to date on the latest treatments.

Second, make sure your second opinion comes from a doctor in a different medical group or hospital from the first. Doctors who know one another or work together often back each other's medical opinions in the interest of maintaining good relations. A couple of good options for second opinions include a National Cancer Institute Comprehensive Cancer Center, a Clinical Cancer Center, or a Community Clinical Oncology Program. To find out if one of these centers is close to you, contact the Cancer Information Service at 1-800-4-CANCER.

Third, take a complete copy of all your medical records from doctor to doctor. Many doctors are quite willing to provide copies of your records although you may have to bear the cost of copies. Even if a doctor isn't willing, you have a legal right to your medical records in most states.

How to take part in a clinical trial

If you are interested in trying an unconventional, unproven treatment for cancer, don't go to a quack who claims to have a secret cure. Instead ask your doctor if you are eligible to participate in a clinical trial.

Researchers use clinical trials to find out if promising new treatment methods really work. If you participate in one of these treatment studies, you (along with others with cancer) will be given the new treatment and carefully watched. All your reactions will be written down and compared with others.

When the study is over, the researchers will gather all their findings, publish them in medical journals, and discuss them at scientific conferences. If the study results are positive, the unconventional experiment you were a part of may become a common treatment for millions of people who have cancer.

If you're interested in participating in a clinical trial, ask your doctor to use PDQ (Physician Data Query) to get information for you. PDQ is a computer database of information from the National Cancer Institute.

You can also call the National Cancer Institute's Information Service to request information about clinical trials. The staff will tell you about cancer-related services in your area. The toll-free number of the Cancer Information Service is 1-800-4-CANCER (1-800-422-6237).

By the way, you don't have to have cancer to take part in a clinical trial. People without cancer can contribute to medical science by helping researchers find new ways to stop the disease before it starts.

Classify your cancer

The possible progression of prostate cancer is determined by looking at the tumor's stage, grade, and volume.

Although classifying cancer is essential to choosing a treatment, it is still a rather controversial process. First, tumors often look remarkably different from one another. Biopsies often don't represent the whole tumor. Second, no grading system currently exists that can reliably predict how deadly a tumor may be or how likely it is that the tumor will respond to treatment. For this reason, researchers continue to try and develop better ways of determining how deadly a tumor may be.

Currently, the most commonly used system to stage prostate cancer is the TNM (Tumor, Nodes, Metastases) system. However, some doctors still use the older Whitmore-Jewett (ABCD) system. A tumor's volume relates closely to its stage.

At this time, the most widely accepted grading system is the Gleason score. In general, the higher the Gleason score, the more cancer that is present. A higher score also suggests that the cancer is likely to progress and metastasize (spread to other parts of the body).

Set the stage for successful treatment

All cancer is not created equal. One type of tumor may lie dormant for years while another is aggressive and deadly. Staging estimates how extensively the disease has grown within or beyond the prostate. Staging is an important part of prostate cancer therapy because the treatment chosen often depends on whether or not the cancer is confined to the gland.

In the beginning, prostate cancer hangs out near the outer edge of the prostate. As the cancer grows, it often penetrates the prostatic capsule (the outer covering of the prostate), moves into nearby tissue, and then spreads to the seminal vesicles. Cancers considered locally advanced have spread into neighboring organs, such as the bladder. Many times prostate cancers have already penetrated the prostatic capsule by the time they are detected.

Stages may range from stage A, where the tumor is still tiny and confined to the prostate, to stage D, where cancer has spread to the lymph nodes or to other organs outside the prostate. The lower the staging, the more likely the cancer can be cured. Stage D tumors are not usually curable.

In the TNM system, T indicates the size and spread of cancer within and near the prostate; N indicates if and where the cancer has spread to the lymph nodes; M indicates that cancer has spread to other organs and sites in the body.

T1 and T2 cancers are confined to the prostate. T1 cancers are usually discovered unexpectedly, such as during surgery for BPH. These cancers cannot be felt during a rectal exam although an elevated PSA may suggest their presence, which a biopsy can then confirm. T2 cancers are often found during a DRE. T3 and T4 cancers have spread from the prostate into surrounding tissues. Cancers classified as N+ indicate the cancer has spread to the lymph nodes. M+ is used for cancers that have spread to other areas in the body.

To see how each stage of cancer affects the prostate, look at Figure 9.1. For a more detailed comparison of the two staging systems, see the chart on page 182.

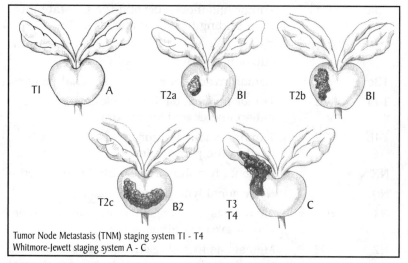

Tumor Node Metastasis (TNM) staging system TI - T4
Whitmore-Jewett staging system A - C

Figure 9.1 - Here you can see the stages of prostate cancer as they are classified by the TNM system and the Whitmore-Jewett staging system. Stages of cancer that have spread to the lymph nodes (N+, DI) and bones (M+, D2) are not shown.

TNM and Jewett-Whitmore staging systems

TNM	Jewett-Whitmore*	Description
TX		Tumor cannot be assessed.
T0		No evidence of tumor.
T1a	A1	Usually found accidentally during TURP for BPH. Biopsy reveals cancer in 5 percent or less of the tissue.
T1b	A2	Usually found accidentally during TURP for BPH. Biopsy reveals cancer in 5 percent or more of the tissue.
T1c	B0	Elevated PSA levels point to the presence of cancer although it still cannot be detected during DRE.
T2a	B1	Tumor involves one-half of a lobe or less.
T2b	B1	Tumor involves more than one-half of a lobe, but not both lobes.
T2c	B2	Tumor involves both lobes.
T3a	C1	Tumor has moved beyond the prostate into surrounding tissue on one side.
T3b	C1	Tumor has moved beyond the prostate into surrounding tissue on both sides.
T3c	C2	Tumor invades one or both seminal vesicles.
T4a	C2	Tumor invades bladder neck and/or external sphincter and/or rectum.
T4b	C2	Tumor invades levator muscles and/or is fixed to the pelvic sidewall.
NX		Regional lymph nodes cannot be assessed.
N0		No regional lymph node metastasis.
N1	D1	Metastasis in a single lymph node, 2 cm or less at greatest dimension.
N2	D1	Metastasis in a single lymph node more than 2 cm, but not more than 5 cm at greatest dimension, or in multiple lymph nodes none more than 5 cm at greatest dimension.

TNM	Jewett-Whitmore*	Description
N3	D1	Metastasis in a lymph node more than 5 cm at greatest dimension.
MX		Presence of distant metastasis cannot be assessed.
M0		No distant metastasis.
M1	D2	Distant metastasis.

*more commonly known as the Whitmore-Jewett staging system

Report on The Management of Clinically Localized Prostate Cancer, The American Urological Association Prostate Cancer Clinical Guidelines Panel, Table 1, 1995, p.13. Copyright 1995, American Urological Association, Inc. Reprinted with permission.

Get a handle on cancer type

Prostate cancer usually begins in the outer portion of the gland. As the tumor grows, the cancer spreads inward. Prostate cancer is considered localized when it is confined totally within the prostate gland. This is stage T1 (A1) or T2 (B1) cancer. Treatment includes watchful waiting, surgery, or radiation therapy.

If the cancer continues to grow, it will eventually spread to local tissues right around the prostate, such as the seminal vesicles. Called locally advanced, this refers to stage T3 (C1) or T4 (C2) cancers. Treatment options may include surgery, radiation, or a combination of treatments.

Cancer that has spread to the lymph nodes or distant organs is considered advanced. Called N+ (D1) or M+ (D2), this type of cancer is generally considered incurable. However, there are treatments that can slow the spread of advanced cancer and may include hormone therapy or experimental approaches. For more information on advanced cancer, see Chapter 11.

Know your enemy: Give your cancer a grade

In order to gauge a tumor's growth potential, doctors usually rely on the Gleason system. Using cell samples obtained during a biopsy, doctors look at the cancer under a microscope to get an idea of how fast the cancer is growing. The system distinguishes progressive grades of prostate cancer based on how well or how poorly the cells are differentiated.

Your Gleason score is measured on a scale of 1 to 5. The pathologist will add the two most common grades together to get a score from 2 to 10. The lower your score, the better.

Cells with distinct, clearly defined borders and clear centers are considered well-differentiated. These cells usually grow the slowest. The inner portions of poorly differentiated cells look gummed together. These cells usually grow the fastest.

Below is a brief description of possible Gleason scores and what they mean.

2,3,4 = Cells are well-differentiated and will probably progress slowly.

5,6,7 = Doctors find it difficult to predict exactly what these cancers will do. However, new evidence suggests that Gleason 5 and 6 tumors progress more slowly than tumors rated 7 or higher.

8,9,10 = Cancer will probably spread quickly.

One of the problems with the Gleason system is that pathologists have trouble distinguishing one grade from another, especially grades 3 and 4. Although this determination is difficult to make, it is extremely important for correctly staging the cancer.

Studies show that metastases rarely occur with grade 3 but often occur with grades 4 and 5. This means that a Gleason score of 6 can be hard to interpret. While a primary grade of 3 and a secondary grade of 3 equaling 6 is a favorable Gleason score, a primary grade of 4 and a secondary grade of 2 equaling 6 or vice versa is not a favorable Gleason score.

The strike zone

About 75 percent of cancers occur in the central and peripheral zones (see Figure 1.2 on page 6). The other 25 percent occur in the transition zone.

A few pointers on ploidy

Sometimes doctors will use a different system from the Gleason scale to grade cancer. Called the ploidy system, this grading scale uses the number of complete chromosome sets in a cell to determine how dangerous or aggressive a cancer may be.

Under the ploidy system, tumor cells may be diploid, tetraploid, or aneuploid. Laboratory tests determine the ploidy of a cancer. Unfortunately, there is not complete agreement on how to interpret ploidy results.

Generally, diploid cancers are considered less aggressive, while aneuploid are thought to be most aggressive. Tetraploid cells fall somewhere in the middle. The ploidy of a cancer can change with time, so your doctor may have you repeat this test.

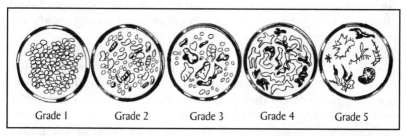

Grade 1   Grade 2   Grade 3   Grade 4   Grade 5

Figure 9.2 - Cancer cells graded on the Gleason scale. Under the Gleason scale, prostate cancer is rated from 1 to 5. One means the cells are well-differentiated; five means the cells are poorly differentiated. The more well-differentiated the cancer cells, the "safer" the cancer is considered to be. The two most common areas of cancer are graded and the two values are added together to obtain an overall score of 2 to 10. Generally, the higher the score, the more dangerous the cancer.

A crash course in classifying cancer

Clinical stage. It's important to understand the difference between clinical stage and pathological stage. Clinical stage is the stage your doctor believes the cancer to be in. He bases his estimation on the results of a variety of tests, which often include the DRE, PSA, TRUS, and a biopsy. For a complete description of these tests, see Chapter 14.

If your doctor uses the TNM system to classify your cancer, he will put a c before TNM to signify that he's classifying your cancer according to clinical stage. For example, a cT2b cancer is thought to be confined to one lobe of your prostate gland based on a clinical classification.

Pathological stage. This is based on a pathologist's examination of actual prostate tissue. Estimating pathological stage used to be possible only after a radical prostatectomy. However, with the development of the Partin tables (see page 187), surgery is no longer necessary to estimate pathological stage.

If your doctor is using the TNM system to classify your cancer according to pathological information, either from an actual examination of prostate tissue or using the Partin tables, he will put a p before TNM to signify that he's classifying your cancer according to pathological stage. If the prostatectomy revealed more or less cancer than the doctor suspected when he gave you the clinical stage, your stage could change. For example, if your clinical findings suggested a cT2b cancer, the pathological findings may point to a pT3 cancer.

Nowadays, doctors can make a much more accurate estimation of pathological stage without surgery, thanks to the development of the Partin tables (named after the Johns Hopkins doctor who created them). These tables combine information from your PSA level, your Gleason score, and your estimated clinical stage (based on the TNM system) to estimate the pathological stage of your cancer. They tell you the likelihood that the cancer is still confined to your prostate or has spread beyond. Knowing whether or not cancer has spread outside the prostate is important in determining which treatment to choose.

These tables are so helpful for choosing a treatment strategy, every urologist should have them posted in his office. Unfortunately, most don't. We've included the Partin tables on the following pages so you can get an idea of the stage of your own cancer before you have to discuss treatment options with your doctor. If you know your PSA level, your Gleason score, and your clinical stage, you can easily find your estimated pathological stage in the following charts.

The easiest way to start your search is with your PSA score. Although the Partin tables are usually considered one chart, we've broken the data down into four tables to make searching easier. Start with chart 1 if you have a PSA score of 0.0-4.0 ng/mL. Go to chart 2 if your PSA is 4.1-10.0 ng/mL. Begin with chart 3 if your PSA levels are between 10.1 and 20 ng/mL. Choose chart 4 if your PSA is greater than 20.0 ng/mL.

For example, if your PSA is 5.8 ng/mL, your clinical stage is T1c, and your Gleason score is 5, you would begin by going to chart 2. Skim across the top of the chart until you find your clinical stage. Now run your finger down the column until you find your appropriate Gleason score (listed in the column to the far left). This tells you that the chance of your prostate cancer being confined to the prostate (called organ-confined disease in the chart) is 71 percent. To find out your chances that the cancer has penetrated the capsule of the prostate, keep your finger in the same column and move down to your Gleason score in the next level (called established capsular penetration). Your risk is 27 percent. A column with a dash (—) and no number indicates researchers didn't have enough information to calculate risk for that particular Gleason score and clinical stage.

Following the same procedure, again move down to the next level. This tells you your risk of seminal vesicle involvement is 2 percent. The last level estimates your risk of lymph node involvement, which in this case is 0 percent.

Partin tables

Chart 1 — PSA 0.0-4.0 ng/mL

Gleason Score	T1a	T1b	Clinical Stage T1c	T2a	T2b	T2c	T3a
Organ-Confined Disease							
2-4	90	80	89	81	72	77	—
5	82	66	81	68	57	62	40
6	78	61	78	64	52	57	35
7	—	43	63	47	34	38	19
8-10	—	31	52	36	24	27	—
Established Capsular Penetration							
2-4	9	19	10	18	25	21	—
5	17	32	18	30	40	34	51
6	19	35	21	34	43	37	53
7	—	44	31	45	51	45	52
8-10	—	43	34	47	48	42	—

Chart 1 — PSA 0.0-4.0 ng/mL (continued)

Gleason			Clinical Stage				
Score	Tla	Tlb	Tlc	T2a	T2b	T2c	T3a
Seminal Vesicle Involvement							
2-4	0	1	1	1	2	2	—
5	1	2	1	2	3	3	7
6	1	2	1	2	3	4	7
7	—	6	4	6	10	12	19
8-10	—	11	9	12	17	21	—
Lymph Node Involvement							
2-4	0	0	0	0	0	0	—
5	0	1	0	0	1	1	2
6	1	2	0	1	2	2	5
7	—	6	1	2	5	5	9
8-10	—	14	4	5	10	10	—

Partin, A.W., et.al, "Combination of Prostate-Specific Antigen, Clinical Stage, and Gleason Score to Predict Pathological Stage of Localized Prostate Cancer," The Journal of the American Medical Association (277,18:1445). Copyright 1997, American Medical Association. Reprinted with permission.

Chart 2 — PSA 4.1-10.0 ng/mL

Gleason			Clinical Stage				
Score	Tla	Tlb	Tlc	T2a	T2b	T2c	T3a
Organ-Confined Disease							
2-4	84	70	83	71	61	66	43
5	72	53	71	55	43	49	27
6	67	47	67	51	38	43	23
7	49	29	49	33	22	25	11
8-10	35	18	37	23	14	15	6
Established Capsular Penetration							
2-4	14	27	15	26	35	29	44
5	25	42	27	41	50	43	57
6	27	44	30	44	52	46	57
7	36	48	40	52	54	48	48
8-10	34	42	40	49	46	40	34

Chart 2 — PSA 4.1-10.0 ng/mL (continued)

Gleason Score	Clinical Stage						
	T1a	T1b	T1c	T2a	T2b	T2c	T3a
Seminal Vesicle Involvement							
2-4	1	2	1	2	4	5	10
5	2	3	2	3	5	6	12
6	2	3	2	3	5	6	11
7	6	9	8	10	15	18	26
8-10	10	15	15	19	24	28	35
Lymph Node Involvement							
2-4	0	1	0	0	1	1	1
5	1	2	0	1	2	2	3
6	3	5	1	2	4	4	9
7	8	12	3	4	9	9	15
8-10	18	23	8	9	16	17	24

Partin, A.W., et.al, "Combination of Prostate-Specific Antigen, Clinical Stage, and Gleason Score to Predict Pathological Stage of Localized Prostate Cancer," The Journal of the American Medical Association (277,18:1445). Copyright 1997, American Medical Association. Reprinted with permission.

Chart 3 — PSA 10.1-20.0 ng/mL

Gleason Score	Clinical Stage						
	T1a	T1b	T1c	T2a	T2b	T2c	T3a
Organ-Confined Disease							
2-4	76	58	75	60	48	53	—
5	61	40	60	43	32	36	18
6	—	33	55	38	26	31	14
7	33	17	35	22	13	15	6
8-10	—	9	23	14	7	8	3
Established Capsular Penetration							
2-4	20	36	22	35	43	37	—
5	33	50	35	50	57	51	59
6	—	49	38	52	57	50	54
7	38	46	45	55	51	45	40
8-10	—	33	40	46	38	33	26

Chart 3 — PSA 10.1-20.0 ng/mL (continued)

Gleason Score	Clinical Stage						
	T1a	T1b	T1c	T2a	T2b	T2c	T3a
Seminal Vesicle Involvement							
2-4	2	4	2	4	7	8	—
5	3	5	3	5	8	9	15
6	—	4	4	5	7	9	14
7	8	11	12	14	18	22	28
8-10	—	15	20	22	25	30	34
Lymph Node Involvement							
2-4	0	2	0	1	1	1	—
5	3	5	1	2	4	4	7
6	—	13	3	4	10	10	18
7	18	24	8	9	17	18	26
8-10	—	40	16	17	29	29	37

Partin, A.W., et.al, "Combination of Prostate-Specific Antigen, Clinical Stage, and Gleason Score to Predict Pathological Stage of Localized Prostate Cancer," The Journal of the American Medical Association (277,18:1445). Copyright 1997, American Medical Association. Reprinted with permission.

Chart 4 — PSA higher than 20.0 ng/mL

Gleason Score	Clinical Stage						
	T1a	T1b	T1c	T2a	T2b	T2c	T3a
Organ-Confined Disease							
2-4	—	38	58	41	29	—	—
5	—	23	40	26	17	19	8
6	—	17	35	22	13	15	6
7	—	—	18	10	5	6	2
8-10	—	3	10	5	3	3	1
Established Capsular Penetration							
2-4	—	47	34	48	52	—	—
5	—	57	48	60	61	55	54
6	—	51	49	60	57	51	46
7	—	—	46	51	43	37	29
8-10	—	24	34	37	28	23	17

Chart 4 — PSA higher than 20.0 ng/mL (continued)

Gleason Score	T1a	T1b	T1c	T2a	T2b	T2c	T3a
Seminal Vesicle Involvement							
2-4	—	9	7	10	14	—	—
5	—	10	9	11	15	19	26
6	—	8	8	10	13	17	21
7	—	—	22	24	27	32	36
8-10	—	20	31	33	33	38	40
Lymph Node Involvement							
2-4	—	4	1	1	3	—	—
5	—	10	3	3	7	7	11
6	—	23	7	8	16	17	26
7	—	—	14	14	25	25	32
8-10	—	51	24	24	36	35	42

Partin, A.W., et.al, "Combination of Prostate-Specific Antigen, Clinical Stage, and Gleason Score to Predict Pathological Stage of Localized Prostate Cancer," The Journal of the American Medical Association (277,18:1445). Copyright 1997, American Medical Association. Reprinted with permission.

The most important phone call you may ever make

Before you settle on a treatment, make sure you've called the National Cancer Institute's Cancer Information Service at 1-800-4-CANCER. Ask them to send you information about the treatment options for your cancer.

At no charge, they will provide you with information on the latest treatment choices for your type and stage of cancer. Also, ask them to check the Physicians Data Query (PDQ) database for information on experimental therapies you may be eligible to try.

Unproven remedies: Should you or shouldn't you?

When you're trying to decide whether to try an unproven remedy, take these steps:

▶ Ask a librarian to help you find out if the treatment has been reported in reputable scientific journals.

▶ Be wary of any treatment that is mainly dietary or nutrition therapy. Scientists don't believe right now that you can get rid of cancerous cells in your body simply by changing your diet.

▶ Watch out for treatments that supposedly have no side effects. Cancer treatments have to be powerful, so it's not likely you'll find an effective therapy without side effects.

Expert help for choosing a treatment

Although the stage of your cancer should affect which treatment you and your doctor choose, it may also depend on which specialist you consult. However, making the choice is a very personal decision because the outcomes of individual treatments are still uncertain at this point.

Urologists tend to recommend surgery while radiation oncologists (cancer specialists) generally advise radiation therapy. In fact, a 1989 survey asking urologists and radiotherapists for treatment recommendations found that 79 percent of the urologists recommended radical prostatectomy while 92 percent of the radiotherapists recommended radiation. Your doctor's recommendations may also depend on the country he practices in. British urologists, for example, tend to recommend watchful waiting.

For these reasons, you may find it helpful to have your family doctor oversee your prostate cancer choice, especially if you feel uncertain about making a decision. Firmly ask each specialist you consult to report his findings and recommendations back to you and your family doctor. This way your family doctor will be in an excellent position to help you sort through and choose an option. Also, if you receive treatment from more than one doctor, it's helpful for your family doctor to monitor all treatments for possible interactions or complications.

Finally, if you're like most men, you'll find it easier to make a decision if you discuss your treatment options with your wife and a trusted friend or minister. It can also be helpful to contact a prostate support group to get feedback on the different options from men who've already made their choice. For more information on finding a support group near you, see Chapter 15.

Rate your overall health to chart your course

When choosing a treatment, you and your doctor should also take into account your overall health. In addition, it's important to realistically assess how many years of life you probably have left. The following questions can help you generate some answers:

- What is your health like generally?

- How old were your parents when they died? What did they die of? (This is important because your parents' life span often influences your own.)

- What is the disease history of your family (high blood pressure, heart problems, diabetes, etc.)?

You want to critically examine your overall health and your expected life span to help you determine how likely you are to benefit from certain treatment options. For example, you may not want to subject your body to the stress of a radical prostatectomy if you expect to live less than 10 years and you have a low-grade cancer.

Generally speaking, the cancer probably won't progress enough to cause you major problems, and you may not live long enough to reap the benefit of surgery. Any side effects, however, will most likely affect you immediately and may lower the quality of the years you do have left.

Working with your doctor, you should be able to make a fairly accurate estimate of your life span. It's important to keep in mind that while your overall health and life span estimate can help you make a choice, it doesn't dictate your decision.

If your estimated life span suggests you won't live long enough to benefit from a radical prostatectomy, but you think you will — go with your gut feeling. Your intuition may be relying on information your conscious mind has missed.

Consider your quality of life

Finally, don't forget to closely examine how different treatments may affect your quality of life. For example, incontinence, impotence, and bowel problems are fairly common side effects of many prostate cancer treatments.

Generally, surgery is more likely to cause sexual and urinary problems while radiation tends to cause more bowel problems. This was brought out in a survey of 274 men who had undergone treatment for prostate cancer one to five years earlier. Among the men, who averaged 70 years old, 70 percent who had surgery reported impotence and 52 percent reported incontinence.

Of the men who chose radiation, 50 percent reported impotence and 15 percent reported incontinence. However, bowel problems are usually more common among men who undergo radiation. In this study, 21 percent of the men who chose radiation reported weekly bouts of diarrhea, while only 8 percent of the men who chose surgery had this problem.

Complications, which some men find more devastating than the cancer itself, may last for years after treatment. Since there is currently no evidence as to whether surgery or radiation is more effective, you may want to at least partly base your treatment decision on which side effects you could live with more easily.

In another study, which compared how quality of life was affected after watchful waiting, radical prostatectomy, or radiation, researchers found that most of the men's daily activities were not compromised no matter which option they chose. In the areas of physical functioning, emotional well-being, energy levels, and overall health, there was not a great deal of difference among the three groups.

Traditional treatment or the road less traveled: Which is right for you?

Traditional wisdom holds that cancer should be treated aggressively. With prostate cancer, this means removing the gland (radical prostatectomy) or bombarding it with radiation. Some experts say these options may offer good prospects for curing the disease if exercised early enough.

If you have a relatively long life expectancy, you may want to seriously consider aggressive treatment. Several studies suggest that prostate cancer is not a harmless disease. In other words, left alone long enough it usually becomes deadly. Currently, prostate cancer is the second leading cause of cancer deaths among men, right behind lung cancer. About 45,000 men in the United States alone die of prostate cancer each year.

Still, others say aggressive treatment does more harm than good. For example, aggressive treatment is often not necessary for men with low-grade tumors (a Gleason score of 2 to 4). Men ages 65 to 75 with low-grade tumors often live just as long as men in the general population.

Also, some experts argue that many of the cancers found in the prostate are too small and insignificant to cause a problem during a man's lifetime. However, other studies show that cancers diagnosed by screening tests such as DRE and PSA are often significant. Most of the cancers found by the DRE and PSA exams do become deadly after a period of 10 to 15 years.

Because prostate cancer is so common among older men — those over age 60 — many of those diagnosed die from other causes before the prostate cancer has time to grow. It has been said that you're more likely to die with prostate cancer than from it.

Get your insurance to pay for your cancer treatment

The issue of whether your insurance company will pay for the cost of your cancer treatment may be the farthest thing from your mind. However, if you don't find out up front, you may face tough times or big bills later.

Once you and your doctor decide on a specific treatment for your cancer, ask him if insurance normally pays for it. Don't panic if he says other patients have had problems. This doesn't necessarily mean the treatment is unsound. For example, some insurance companies and HMOs resist paying for bone marrow transplants on the grounds they are experimental.

Even more disturbing is that most insurance companies and HMOs who deny coverage have no clearly written guidelines for doing so. By all appearances, they vary their decisions in a totally arbitrary manner from case to case.

Your first step should be to have your doctor call the insurance company and request a predetermination, approval from the insurance company that allows you to go ahead and receive treatment. Once they grant approval, they agree to pay whatever portion of that treatment is covered by your policy.

If your insurance company balks, start preparing the papers you'll need to convince them otherwise. This probably will include getting a second opinion on your need for the treatment. You'll also want to ask the insurance company what other papers they need in order to reconsider their decision.

Some other good sources of advice may include local cancer groups and the National Coalition for Cancer Survivorship. This organization offers practical advice and help for people with cancer having insurance problems. You can reach them at (301) 585-2626.

If your insurance company stubbornly refuses to budge, bring out the big guns. Ask your doctor if he can recommend a lawyer who's dealt with similar problems before. If your doctor believes the treatment is the best medical choice for you, and the lawyer can make a good case, most insurance companies will pay up.

Vital information on treatment options

Watchful waiting

For older men with early-stage prostate cancer, a number of doctors are dispensing a different kind of advice: Wait and see. Generally, the ideal watchful-waiting candidate is a man with a stage A or B tumor, a low Gleason score, a low PSA, and a relatively short life expectancy. However, anyone can choose watchful waiting if they want to avoid the side effects of other forms of therapy.

A popular option in Europe, more and more men are choosing watchful waiting since PSA tests have made early detection possible. Monitoring your condition regularly is also easier and more accurate with PSA testing. The downside of watchful waiting is that tumors can sometimes grow rapidly, and by the time you make the decision to treat aggressively, it could be too late.

Doctors are clearly divided on its merits, but this "watchful waiting" philosophy got a boost recently by a report in *The New England Journal of Medicine*. The study analyzed case records of 828 prostate cancer patients treated conservatively (watchful waiting or hormone treatments but no surgery or radiation therapy).

It found that 10 years after diagnosis, 87 percent of those with slow-growing, localized prostate tumors were still alive.

Of those diagnosed with more aggressive cancer, 34 percent remained alive at the 10-year mark. Supporters say watchful waiting is a practical alternative for men in their late 60s or older, whose life spans may be limited by advanced age and serious ailments such as heart disease. If treated, these men could suffer the trauma and adverse effects of cancer therapy with little or no benefit.

However, if you are in relatively good health with the prospect of quite a few good years ahead of you, there's another side to watchful waiting you may want to consider. First, given enough time even small, well-differentiated prostate cancers tend to progress into larger, less well-differentiated and more aggressive tumors, which are harder to cure and more likely to kill. In fact, one recent study found that low-grade tumors have a 55 percent chance of causing death within 15 years. Those studies that suggest most men do not die of prostate cancer but with it include men who are at high risk of dying from other causes and who generally have less aggressive forms of the cancer.

Even if you initially chose watchful waiting, you are free to choose any other treatment at any time. In the meantime, the progress of your tumor will still be monitored. How often you need to be monitored will depend on the stage of your cancer and on your general health. If you develop symptoms, you will be given treatment for those symptoms. However, that treatment is not intended to cure the cancer.

Men most likely to benefit from watchful waiting

- Have a shorter life expectancy, usually 10 years or less.

- Have a PSA level of 10 ng/mL or less, a Gleason score of 2 to 4, and a tumor that is undetectable by DRE.

Pros

▶ Low treatment cost, especially during early stages of cancer. If a tumor doesn't progress much during your lifetime, costs may remain low. However, they may rise significantly if other treatment interventions are required. Treatment for a case of metastatic prostate cancer can cost $70,000 or more.

▶ No side effects associated with treatment.

▶ Fairly good 10-year survival rate. Men with tumors that are well to moderately differentiated have a fairly good chance of surviving for at least 10 years.

Cons

▶ Cancer is more likely to progress and become incurable.

▶ Complications related to the tumor may end up reducing your quality of life. Possible complications include pain, problems with urination, anemia, bone fractures, blood clots, spinal cord compression, and paralysis.

▶ Continued anxiety about doing nothing to stop cancer progression. This in itself may take a heavy toll on your health.

Nature's own healers

If you've opted for watchful waiting, you may be interested to know that several more natural therapies are being studied to see if they can help with prostate cancer. Some of the studies look promising. Since many of the side effects of these treatments are few or mild, you may want to consider trying them. See Chapter 10 for more information on these treatments as well as tips on natural ways you can set your body's own healing forces in motion.

Surgery

Radical prostatectomy

Also called open prostatectomy, this is a major surgery that removes the entire prostate. Radical prostatectomy is most effective if the cancer is still confined to the prostate gland.

A surgeon can take two possible approaches to a radical prostatectomy:

▶ **Retropubic radical prostatectomy** — The most common type of radical prostatectomy, this surgery involves making a cut in the lower abdomen behind the pubic bone (retropubic) to reach the prostate.

▶ **Perineal radical prostatectomy** — In this approach, the surgeon goes through the perineal region (the area between the scrotum and the anus) to reach the prostate. This is generally considered to be a less strenuous surgery so it may be used in older men or in men with poorer health who may have higher risks of complications.

The nerve-sparing prostate surgery, which attempts to preserve sexual potency, is typically performed during the retropubic radical prostatectomy. (Sometimes a nerve-sparing surgery is attempted during a perineal radical prostatectomy.) Unless the nerve-sparing procedure is performed, which preserves the ability to have erections in up to 70 to 90 percent of men, surgery will generally cause impotence.

Typically, once the surgeon has cut into the area to begin removing the prostate, he will take a lymph node sample from the area nearest the prostate. He will immediately send this sample to the lab to be examined for cancer. If cancer is found, he will often stop the surgery immediately and stitch you back up, feeling there is no need to remove the prostate since cancer has already spread. If the lymph nodes are cancer free, he will proceed.

Once the surgeon identifies the prostate, he begins the process of cutting it loose from surrounding tissue. The last step in removing the prostate involves detaching it from the bladder. The seminal vesicles come out with the prostate.

Because the prostate and bladder are attached to each other, the surgeon must cut a hole in the bottom of the bladder about the size of a quarter. Using stitches, the surgeon shrinks the hole to about the size of a dime. Then he pulls the bladder and urethra close and stitches them together.

Once the body heals, urine will run from the bladder straight into the urethra instead of going through the part of the urethra that passed through the prostate (the prostatic urethra) as it did before. The surgery usually takes between two to four hours.

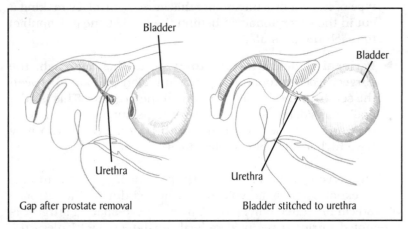

Figure 9.3 - Once the prostate is removed, there is a gap between the urethra and the bladder. To give urine a way out of the body, the urethra is stitched to the bladder.

Recent advances in surgical technique for radical prostatectomy appear to have reduced the risk of complications. A better understanding of prostate anatomy and better ways of viewing the prostate during surgery allow surgeons to operate more carefully. This means less blood loss and less risk of incontinence and impotence after surgery. Hospital stay has also been significantly reduced. Most men now only need to stay from three to six days.

However, complications still occur. These include bleeding, which may require a transfusion, and the risk of infection that often accompanies transfusion. (See Chapter 6 for more information on transfusion.) You may also have difficulty with the connection the surgeon created between the bladder neck and urethra, as well as rectal injury.

You will probably experience incontinence after surgery, which may or may not be temporary. Incontinence occurs because of damage to the urethral sphincter, sometimes called the "gatekeeper of urinary flow." Your risk of incontinence depends on both your anatomy and on the skill and experience of your surgeon.

In order to allow the new connection between your bladder and urethra to heal, you will leave the hospital with a Foley catheter in place (see illustration 6.1 on page 135). This will normally be removed two to three weeks after surgery. Most men are incontinent immediately after removal of the catheter so it's important to take an adult diaper with you the day you expect to have the catheter removed.

Although many men do eventually regain urinary control, it's impossible to predict how long that might take. It can vary from several weeks to up to a year. Three months after surgery about half the men will have regained control. For tips on dealing with incontinence, see Chapter 12.

Most men either suffer from total incontinence, which is a complete inability to control urine, or stress incontinence, which is urine leakage triggered by coughing, sneezing, or straining.

Nerve-sparing radical prostatectomy

At one time, surgeons made a wide swath around the prostate, removing most of the surrounding nerves and leaving most men impotent or incontinent or both.

This is changing, however, thanks to pioneering research done in the 1980s by Dr. Patrick Walsh, urologist-in-chief at Johns Hopkins University Medical Center and professor at Johns Hopkins School of Medicine.

With the development of the Walsh technique, surgeons began cutting closer to the prostate, taking care to spare nearby nerves, which greatly reduces the risk of impotence. If the doctor is concerned that the cancer may have spread right outside the prostate or he's not interested in preserving sexual potency, he will simply remove these nerves with the rest of the prostate.

Unfortunately, the older you are, the less likely that this procedure will be effective. Up to 70 to 90 percent of men age 50 or younger are likely to retain potency with this procedure while only 25 percent of men over 70 retain potency. About 58 percent of men age 60 to 70 retain potency.

The nerve-sparing prostatectomy also helps preserve the function of the urethral sphincter, which controls urine flow. This means less of a risk of incontinence following surgery.

However, a recent study has suggested that the nerve-sparing procedure may not work as well as researchers had hoped. In a small study of 94 men, Boston researchers found that most men who had either a nerve-sparing or a non-nerve-sparing radical prostatectomy were impotent one year later. Surprisingly, they also found that the men who underwent the nerve-sparing procedure had more trouble with incontinence than men who underwent the non-nerve-sparing surgery.

Still, other experts, including Dr. Walsh, contend that the procedure is effective when performed correctly. He suggests that if you wish to have a successful nerve-sparing prostatectomy, you should seek the services of an experienced surgeon working at an expert center.

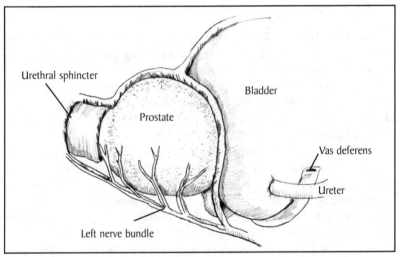

Figure 9.4 - Nerve-sparing radical prostatectomy. If the cancer has not invaded the prostate wall, your surgeon may be able to preserve your sexual potency by carefully separating nerve bundles from the left and right sides of your prostate. This technique was pioneered by Dr. Patrick Walsh of Johns Hopkins University and is known as the nerve-sparing radical prostatectomy.

In addition, Dr. Walsh and others are currently testing an electronic device, which may make it easier for all surgeons to perform nerve-sparing prostatectomies. It helps determine the location of nerves that are essential for erections. Approval from the FDA looks promising.

Regardless, other doctors and even prostate cancer survivors remain skeptical of the effectiveness of the Walsh technique. The national director of the support organization US TOO notes that while doctors may be learning more about how to protect those vital nerve bundles, very few can perform the surgery successfully. Some doctors even go so far as to warn men not to expect normal erections if they choose surgery.

Even with the nerve-sparing prostatectomy, there is still a significant risk of permanent impotence. Generally, your risk of impotence is directly related to your age and the extent of your tumor. The older you are and the more extensive your tumor, the more likely surgery will leave you impotent. For men who do regain the ability to have an erection, it may be a gradual process, taking from six to 12 months. For practical solutions to impotence, see Chapter 13.

Recently, there has been some concern that surgery for prostate cancer may cause cancerous cells to spread through the bloodstream. In response to this concern, researchers have noted that using drugs to shut down the production of testosterone (called neoadjuvant hormone therapy) can prevent potential cancer spread. Ask your doctor if he thinks this would be beneficial for you. For more on neoadjuvant hormone therapy, see page 213.

After a radical prostatectomy, your PSA levels should fall to around zero. An elevated PSA level after surgery suggests some cancer may still be present or has recurred. This means the cancer may continue to progress. PSA levels may rise in 27 to 53 percent of the men who undergo radical prostatectomy.

In order to prevent progression, researchers have been investigating radiation after prostatectomy as a possible treatment. It appears to do the trick, especially in men whose PSA levels are 2 ng/mL or less.

Wayne State University researchers found that 83 percent of men who had PSA levels of 2 ng/mL or less showed no evidence of cancer progression during a follow-up period of at least a year and a half. Only 33 percent of those men whose PSA levels were higher showed no disease progression.

If you decide radiation after surgery is the route you should take, keep in mind the possible side effects that may develop from radiation. These may include urinary problems, nausea, vomiting, diarrhea, and impotence. The good news is that a recent study from Belgium found that radiation after surgery does not appear to increase the risk of incontinence.

As more cancers are found at an early stage, the need for additional treatment after prostatectomy should decrease.

Men most likely to benefit from radical prostatectomy

- Have a relatively long life expectancy.

- Surgery is their preferred treatment option.

- Have no major health conditions that might rule out surgery.

Pros

▶ May be able to completely remove cancer and totally cure some men. Even in men who aren't cured, the surgery may be able to slow the cancer's progression significantly.

Cons

▶ Cancer not always totally removed and may progress.

▶ Incontinence. Rates of incontinence following radical prostatectomy range from 4 percent to 50 percent for stress incontinence and from 0 percent to 15.4 percent for severe incontinence. Total incontinence is low in men who are younger than 70 at the time of surgery.

▶ Impotence. 30 to 90 percent of men may experience impotence after a radical prostatectomy.

▶ Death. Although the risk is low, ranging from 0 to 5 percent, it does increase with age. Studies show a 1.4 percent risk in men ages 75 to 80 and a 4.6 percent risk for men ages 80 and older.

Pull the plug on unnecessary surgeries

Despite advances in technology, doctors still have problems accurately predicting the spread of prostate cancer. Neither transrectal ultrasound, magnetic resonance imaging (MRI), nor a computed tomography (CT or CAT) scan can predict with reliable accuracy whether or not the cancer has metastasized (spread) beyond the prostate. This means some men suffer the trauma and side effects of a radical prostatectomy only to find out several years later that the very problem they were trying to avoid — the spread of cancer — has occurred anyway.

However, doctors now have a new diagnostic tool at their disposal that promises to make many of these unnecessary surgeries a problem of the past. Called prostascint, this test can accurately detect cancer spread outside the prostate.

Approved by the FDA in 1996, prostascint works by way of antibodies that attach themselves to the walls of prostate cancer cells. A harmless radioactive particle, designed to show up during a whole-body scan, is attached to the antibody.

A man to be tested with prostascint is given an injection and told to return four days later for a whole-body scan, which will then reveal the exact location of all prostate cancer in the body.

For prostate cancer that is definitely confined to the prostate, most doctors recommend a radical prostatectomy. If the cancer has spread to lymph nodes in the pelvis, radiation and/or hormone therapy may be the best option. For prostate cancer that has spread beyond the lymph nodes into other areas of the body, hormone therapy is usually recommended.

---

2 types of prostatectomy

A prostatectomy for BPH is quite different from a prostatectomy for prostate cancer. A prostatectomy for BPH removes all the tissue inside the prostate, leaving only the prostatic capsule. It's like a sack with no groceries inside. A prostatectomy for prostate cancer removes the entire prostate. You have neither sack nor groceries left. See figure 5.6 on page 107.

When surgery may offer you a better chance of survival

In a new study of 3,626 men, researchers provide updated estimates of survival rates after radical prostatectomy. Unlike previous studies that suggested survival rates differed depending on where you lived, this study found no such difference.

For men age 65 or younger with well-differentiated to moderately differentiated cancers, the survival rate following surgery was 75 to 97 percent. For men age 65 or younger with poorly differentiated cancers, the survival rate was 60 to 75 percent.

For men older than 65 with well-differentiated to moderately differentiated cancers, the survival rate following surgery was 82 to 95 percent. For men older than 65 with poorly differentiated cancers, the survival rate was 70 to 86 percent.

While these studies offer more insight into the survival rates for radical prostatectomy, the researchers caution against comparing these percentages with other treatment methods, such as radiation and watchful waiting. Because this study concerned itself only with surgery and based its ratings on pathological staging, it cannot be used to draw conclusions from other treatment methods, which typically rely on clinical staging.

In addition, although this study may offer hope to men who aren't comfortable with watchful waiting, it doesn't address the issue of which men might have done just as well without surgery.

When surgery alone is not enough

Some doctors tend to downplay the risk of side effects or the need for additional treatment in the interest of helping you live longer. However, if you're as concerned about the quality of your life as the quantity of it, tell your doctor to be up-front with you about risks of side effects and the need for retreatment.

Reports that radical prostatectomy rarely requires additional treatment may have misled many men into believing that a radical prostatectomy alone will provide effective management for their prostate cancer. However, this is not necessarily the case.

According to a recent study of more than 3,000 men on Medicare, about one-third of the men who undergo a radical prostatectomy may need additional treatment within five years. About 35 percent of the men had to undergo hormone therapy or have their testicles removed within five years of surgery.

One reason for this relatively high rate of retreatment is that during surgery doctors discovered that almost half of the men thought to have cancer confined to their prostates did not. Cancer that has moved beyond the prostate almost always requires treatment besides surgery to stop or slow its spread.

As newer and better systems are developed to help doctors more accurately stage cancer, the need for retreatment after surgery should decrease. Until then, you may find it helpful to know that for men with cancer supposedly confined to their prostates, the risk of requiring retreatment within five years ranged from 15.6 percent for well-differentiated cancer to 41.5 percent for poorly differentiated cancer.

For cancer that had moved beyond the prostate into nearby tissue, the risk of needing retreatment ranged from 22.7 percent for well-differentiated cancer to 68.1 percent for poorly differentiated cancer.

Knowing this may mean that you choose a different course of therapy or that you simply prepare yourself for the possibility that additional treatment may be necessary.

How radiation kills cancer cells

Radiation attempts to stop the progress of prostate cancer by interfering with cancer cell reproduction. Radiation is a good option for men when the cancer has penetrated the prostatic capsule but has only spread to surrounding tissue. It's also a good choice for older men who may not hold up well under surgery. Generally, however, men most likely to get the best results from external beam radiotherapy are also ideal candidates for radical prostatectomy.

Typically, 40 to 70 percent of men retain their ability to have an erection after radiation treatment. Generally, younger, more sexually active, men are likely to remain potent. If impotence does occur, it may take months to a year before it becomes apparent. Whereas impotence from surgery usually involves nerve damage, radiation-induced impotence is usually caused by scarring and blocking of penile veins, which may take at least six months to begin.

There are two basic types of radiation:

External beam radiation. This type of radiation therapy bombards the general vicinity of the prostate in order to destroy the cancer cells. It causes fewer side effects than surgery, but it may be less effective.

A new twist on external beam radiation called 3-D conformal radiation uses 3-D images and computers to direct delivery of the radiation. This allows the radiation beam to be targeted more precisely at the prostate and seminal vesicles, which means less damage to surrounding tissues. Doctors hope this also means fewer side effects and complications.

Although doctors using conformal radiation say cure rates are similar to surgery, men who choose this treatment have not been followed for as long as men who choose surgery.

External radiation will mean five-day-a-week treatments (which usually take about 10 minutes) for seven or eight weeks. This treatment normally won't interfere with any of your usual activities. Side effects may include weakness, diarrhea, blood in the stool, nausea, and vomiting. Generally, however, this treatment is well-tolerated, and the irritating symptoms will go away within two weeks to two months after the end of treatment.

After radiation treatment, your PSA levels should drop into the low-normal range. About 14 to 36 percent of the men who undergo radiation will eventually experience rising PSA levels.

Interstitial radiation (also called brachytherapy). This is a newer version of radiation that may increase radiation's effectiveness if used in addition to external beam radiation. If used alone, it also appears to have a good success rate with a smaller risk of side effects. However, few long-term studies have been done using this approach, so long-term outcome is unknown.

During this procedure, a man is placed under general or spinal anesthesia while 80 to 120 radioactive seeds (usually iodine 125 or palladium 103) are implanted into his prostate. Using ultrasound for guidance, the radiologist uses long, hollow needles inserted through the perineum to place the seeds in a precise geometric arrangement.

Seeds are left in place permanently and continue to emit low levels of radiation for several months. Although the risk is probably small, just to be on the safe side you shouldn't let small children or pregnant women sit on your lap for several months afterward. Your radiologist will be able to give you more specific guidelines. Side effects may include painful urination for a couple of months after implantation.

This 60- to 90-minute procedure is usually performed on an outpatient basis although it may require a one-night stay. Although follow-up time for this procedure is limited to seven years currently, the success rates look promising, ranging from 92 percent cure rate for milder cancers to a 73 percent cure rate for more aggressive cancers. However, more follow-up needs to be done before this figure can be considered dependable or the true outcome of the procedure is known.

Other researchers are openly skeptical of brachytherapy, saying the results are exaggerated. They claim that the increase in the number of procedures being done is driven by a desire to make money, both by manufacturers and doctors. You may generally find that a number of doctors prefer surgery over radiation, especially surgeons. Dr. Steven N. Rous, author of *The Prostate Book*, explains. "My own bias in favor of surgical treatment reflects, in part, the fact that I am a surgeon; but I would also like to think that it reflects my very genuine belief that the cure rate and long-term survival without any evidence of any remaining cancer is significantly better with surgical treatment."

However, a decided plus of brachytherapy is that PSA levels seem much less inclined to rise after this treatment. In a follow-up of 291 men who underwent brachytherapy, rising PSAs were detected in only 14. However, longer-term studies of more men are needed to confirm this finding as well.

You may want to consider another treatment besides brachytherapy if you've undergone TURP for BPH. Men undergoing brachytherapy who've previously had TURP or a severe urinary tract disease tend to have a much higher rate of urinary complications. Also, if you have either a high-grade tumor or a large tumor, you are not a good candidate for brachytherapy.

Sometimes treatment involves a combination of both external and interstitial radiation. While brachytherapy works to eliminate cancer within the prostate, external beam radiation helps destroy cancer cells that may have moved beyond the prostate.

Because the pros and cons for external beam radiation and brachytherapy differ slightly, they're listed separately below.

Men most likely to benefit from radiation

- Have a PSA level below 20 ng/mL and a low-stage, low-grade tumor.

- Have a relatively long life expectancy.

- Those over 70 who may not be able to hold up well under surgery or men with serious medical conditions that may rule out surgery.

- Radiation is their preferred treatment option.

- Have no significant risk factors that rule out radiation. For example, hip replacements can significantly interfere with the delivery of radiation. Also, if you have lupus or other similar conditions, an inflammatory bowel disease, or previous prostate or abdominal surgery, you will probably not qualify for radiation therapy. This treatment is probably also not in your best interest if the cancer has spread to your lymph nodes.

External beam radiation

Pros

▶ Fairly well tolerated as long as most modern techniques are used.

▶ May be able to totally cure some men.

▶ Death is rare.

Cons

▶ The prostate is not removed, which means the cancer may be able to persist and progress.

▶ Depending on your age and the quality of your erections before treatment, you have about a 30 to 66 percent chance of becoming impotent after treatment.

▶ Approximately 2 to 9 percent of men become incontinent following radiation.

▶ About 3 percent of men develop chronic bowel problems following external beam radiation.

Brachytherapy (interstitial radiotherapy)

Pros

▶ Very convenient technique. The procedure is usually performed on an outpatient basis. There is some soreness, but not usually a great deal of pain afterward.

▶ No need for weekly radiation treatments.

Cons

▶ This may be an inferior method of controlling localized tumors.

▶ Treatment may fail in 5 to 10 years.

▶ More follow-up needs to be done before this treatment can be sufficiently evaluated.

▶ The risk of impotence ranges from 20 to 25 percent, especially in men younger than 70. For men over 70, the rate rises to 50 percent.

▶ Persistent bowel or urinary problems affect a small number of men. There is a less than 1 percent risk of incontinence.

Update on prostate cancer treatments

In a recent comparison of prostate cancer treatments, researchers found that the benefits of some treatments had been overestimated while others had been underestimated.

Most men who are about to undergo radical prostatectomy have their lymph nodes checked for cancer first. If cancer is present, the surgery is often canceled. However, men who are treated with watchful waiting or radiation therapy usually do not have their lymph nodes checked for cancer.

Because no lymph node check is performed (and there is currently no other method that is 100 percent reliable in detecting the spread of cancer), many men who choose watchful waiting or radiation have their cancers understaged. What this means is that many times these men's cancers may be more advanced than they appear, making their treatment choice of watchful waiting or radiation look less effective than a radical prostatectomy.

To overcome this bias, these researchers took a different approach to the data. After following nearly 60,000 men with localized prostate cancer for 10 years, the researchers came up with some new findings about the different treatment options.

Men with low-grade cancer have generally high 10-year survival rates despite their treatment choice — 90 to 94 percent hung in there. Previous estimates weren't too far off — they found men survived 89 to 98 percent of the time despite treatment choice.

Among men with medium-grade cancers, 87 percent survived 10 years after radical prostatectomy; 76 percent survived 10 years after radiation therapy; and 77 percent survived 10 years of watchful waiting.

Previous estimates of survival rates found 91 percent of men to survive 10 years after radical prostatectomy; 74 percent survived 10 years after radiation therapy; and 76 percent survived 10 years of watchful waiting.

Among men with high-grade cancers, 67 percent survived 10 years after radical prostatectomy; 53 percent survived 10 years after radiation therapy; and 45 percent survived 10 years of watchful waiting. Previous estimates of survival rates found 76 percent to survive 10 years after a radical prostatectomy; 52 percent for radiation treatment; and 43 percent survived 10 years of watchful waiting.

Hormone therapy to slow the spread

Generally, the spread of prostate cancer is dependent on male sex hormones (androgens), especially testosterone. Reducing androgen levels will usually shrink or slow the progression of prostate cancer — sometimes dramatically.

There are two basic ways to lower male hormone levels:

- by surgically removing the testicles (orchiectomy)

- by using drugs that prevent the release or interfere with the action of these hormones, such as luteinizing hormone releasing hormone (LHRH) agonists, anti-androgens, or a combination of these drugs.

Hormone therapy usually causes a loss of sexual desire and impotence. Some men also experience hot flashes, night sweats, depression, and mood swings.

Although hormone treatment is generally used to treat advanced (metastatic) cases of prostate cancer, it is sometimes used to reduce the size of a tumor (often referred to as downstaging) before a radical prostatectomy or radiation therapy.

Neoadjuvant hormone therapy

In the past, hormone therapy has been used mainly to relieve pain and slow the progression of advanced prostate cancer. However, recently some doctors have begun to use neoadjuvant hormone therapy in an attempt to downstage cancer.

Recent research suggests that using hormone therapy for two to six months before a radical prostatectomy or radiation may lead to more complete removal of the cancer. Some researchers also suggest neoadjuvant hormone therapy can be used to reduce the risk that surgery may cause cancer cells to spread further.

Researchers theorize that if as many cancer cells as possible are eliminated with hormones before the main treatment begins, then getting rid of the rest of the cancer cells by surgery or radiation will be easier. Although hormone therapy does cause the tumor to shrink and PSA levels to fall, there is no evidence that cancer that has escaped from the prostate can be forced back inside, so that removing it becomes more likely.

Whether this approach offers any real benefit or not is unclear. Although some studies look promising, early results show no improvement in the number of men whose PSA rises after surgery, a possible sign cancer is still present or has recurred.

Another possible drawback is that using hormone therapy before surgery makes it more difficult to perform the nerve-sparing prostatectomy. It also makes it more difficult to truly determine how far the prostate cancer has spread.

Generally, neoadjuvant hormone therapy is reserved for men with locally advanced cancer (cancer that has spread into tissue right outside the prostate). If you're interested in this approach, ask your doctor if you could benefit. For more information on hormone treatment for advanced cancer, see Chapter 11.

Combinations for more effective treatment

Sometimes your doctor may suggest a combination of surgery, radiation and/or hormone therapy. Ask questions about possible risks and benefits of each type of treatment, including combination therapy, so you can choose the treatment that seems best for you.

Several recent studies provide support for combination treatments. In a study of 800 men ages 51 to 80 with prostate cancer, researchers at the University of Toronto found a 17 percent higher five-year survival rate for men treated with both radiation and goserelin, a hormone that inhibits testosterone production.

Experimental treatments

Cryosurgery

Also called cryosurgical ablation of the prostate (CSAP) or cryotherapy, this "ice cube" surgery attempts to eliminate cancer by freezing the cells to death.

To perform this procedure, small cuts are made in the perineal area. Guided by ultrasound, probes filled with liquid nitrogen are positioned around the prostate. Liquid nitrogen flowing through the probes is then used to freeze the entire prostate and usually the surrounding tissue as well.

To avoid damaging the urethra by freezing, a transurethral warming coil is used to protect it. However, this may also preserve a little prostate tissue near the urethra, which opens up the possibility that some cancer cells may remain there and eventually spread.

This surgery usually takes two to three hours. You should be able to go home either the same day or the next day. The most common side effects are urinary retention and perineal pain although incontinence and impotence are also fairly common. You will need to wear a catheter for 10 to 14 days.

If you experience continued perineal pain, nonsteroidal anti-inflammatory drugs (NSAIDs) and sitz baths (sitting for 15 minutes in a few inches of hot water) may offer relief. Be sure to let your doctor know that your pain is ongoing. He may recommend periodic catheterization or a short course of steroids.

If this treatment sounds interesting to you, keep in mind that the effectiveness of this method has not yet been established, and it continues to be studied. Reports note that after surgery up to 56 to 59 percent of men undergoing this procedure have detectable PSA levels, which suggest cancer is still present or has recurred.

Some studies report rates of impotence after cryosurgery to be as high as 50 percent. This procedure may also cause urinary incontinence. Overall, the complication rate for cryosurgery is about 10 percent. However, long-term complications and results are not known.

One study found a significantly lower risk of complications in men with prostate glands smaller than 30 grams. These findings support the "downsizing" of larger glands using neoadjuvant hormone therapy for several months before cryosurgery.

Because cryotherapy is considered experimental, experts suggest that men who wish to try this therapy seek treatment at a medical university or other institution that is committed to scientifically developing the procedure.

Men most likely to benefit from cryosurgery

- Appears to be an effective treatment for men who do not respond well to local radiation.

Pros

▶ Cryosurgery is easier on the body than radical prostatectomy. There is generally less blood loss, so you're less likely to need a transfusion. You'll also have less pain because no major incision is made to perform cryosurgery.

▶ Can be performed on an outpatient basis. Sometimes a one-night stay is required.

▶ The procedure can be repeated if not all the cancer was removed the first time. Also, trying cryosurgery does not make you ineligible to try other procedures, including external beam radiation or radical prostatectomy. However, brachytherapy is no longer possible.

Cons

▶ No long-term follow-up information available on the outcome and risk of complications for cryotherapy. Currently, researchers have only followed men who have undergone cryotherapy using current methods for about three years.

▶ Risk of impotence is about 45 percent.

▶ Risk of incontinence is around 10 percent.

▶ Formations of fistulas (unnatural openings) between the urethra and the rectum. The risk of fistula development is around 2 percent. Fistulas can cause urinary incontinence or infection. In fact, repeated urinary tract infections do tend to be a problem with cryosurgery. Although some fistulas will close on their own, most need to be repaired surgically.

▶ Because cryosurgery is considered experimental, it may not be covered by your insurance.

Resist recurrent cancer

To monitor for cancer recurrence, it's important to have your PSA levels tested regularly. You should also have a regular digital rectal exam.

Although there is no set standard for monitoring cancer recurrence, most doctors test PSA levels every three to six months following treatment for the first one to two years, then move to an annual testing schedule.

In men who've had a radical prostatectomy, PSA levels should be undetectable no more than three months after surgery. For men who chose radiation, their PSA levels should continue to fall until reaching a final low point after about a year. At that point, the PSA should be 1 ng/mL or less.

However, you should keep in mind that PSA varies and that other aspects of life besides the presence or absence of cancer can affect these levels. A series of high levels doesn't always point to cancer just as a series of low levels does not always signal the absence of cancer.

If cancer has recurred after surgery, the most common treatment is radiation. If cancer recurs after radiation, surgery or cryotherapy are options.

Give your health the marriage boost

Some men might joke that marriage is a ball-and-chain event — that their freedom ended when they said "I do." It may be a matter of opinion whether marriage does indeed end your freedom, but it's a statistical fact that it may prolong your life.

One study of men with prostate cancer found that married men survive longer than single, widowed, or divorced men. Married men had a median survival rate of 69 months, almost double the 38 months for men who were separated or widowed. Men who had never been married had a median survival rate of 49 months, and the rate for divorced men was 55 months.

That extra time could be a result of married men detecting their cancer earlier because their wives encourage them to go to the doctor. However, researchers think it is more likely that support from a loving spouse can ease some of the stress and depression felt by a cancer patient. Too much stress can shorten life spans, even for people without cancer.

Another study found that the partners of men with prostate cancer felt more psychological distress than the patients did. Sharing the burden can both increase your life and strengthen your relationship.

According to Pete Wilson, a prostate cancer survivor, not sharing the burden can end your relationship. "We're getting divorced, partly because of the way I handled PCa [prostate cancer] with my wife — I was very closed in, secretive, did all the research myself, and so on. Left her out of the picture entirely, which was not good for her. I didn't do it purposely, of course, but I think it takes conscious effort to involve a spouse the way she'd like to be involved."

In other words, talk to your wife, don't shut her out. Share the burden. Your cancer affects her, too, and she may be able to help buy you some more precious, healthy time.

The future looks bright

Though prostate cancer research has yielded significant advancements in the last decade, there's still a long way to go, says FDA's Max Robinowitz, M.D., medical officer in FDA's Center for Devices and Radiological Health. "The dilemmas [of treatment] are due to the power of the cancer and the limits to our current knowledge and therapies," he says.

Still, men have made rapid strides in the past few years by openly acknowledging their struggle with prostate cancer and demanding newer and more effective treatments. With the interest that's been generated, more scientists and doctors are working harder to meet men's demands. A day rarely goes by without a new study coming out, and each one is another step toward more effective treatment and an eventual cure.

In summary

Although a diagnosis of cancer is frightening, it's far from being a death sentence. Becoming informed is the first step in your fight against prostate cancer.

It's important that you ask your doctor enough questions to clearly understand it. Find out how he diagnosed the cancer, how likely it is to spread, what the stage and grade of your cancer is, and what your treatment options are. Write down the answers.

Now is the time to seek a second opinion. Both the length and quality of your life may be at stake, so it's important to make sure you've explored all possible options. You also need to be sure you've found the medical team that will best meet your needs.

Your next step is to understand the stage and grade of your cancer. This information is essential in helping you and your doctor choose a treatment option. Staging estimates how extensively the disease has grown within or beyond the prostate. The stage may be determined by a variety of different tests, such as the DRE, PSA, biopsy, or by a combination of these tests.

In order to gauge how fast a cancer is likely to grow, doctors usually rely on the Gleason system. Using cell samples obtained during a biopsy, doctors look at the cancer under a microscope to get an idea of how fast the cancer is growing. The system distinguishes progressive grades of prostate cancer based on how well or how poorly the cells are differentiated.

Once your doctor has determined the stage and grade of your cancer, you're almost ready to begin considering treatment options. First, be sure to see the Partin Tables beginning on page 187. These tables combine information from your PSA level, your Gleason score, and the stage of your cancer. They will help you determine the likelihood that the cancer is still confined to your prostate or has spread beyond. Knowing whether or not cancer has spread outside the prostate is very helpful in determining which treatment option to choose.

Unfortunately, choosing a treatment remains one of the most controversial and difficult issues to deal with after a diagnosis of prostate cancer. When making a choice, it's important to consider both your overall health and your quality of life. Basically, you have three options: watchful waiting, radical prostatectomy, and radiation therapy.

Because making a choice can be so difficult, you may find it helpful to have your family doctor oversee your prostate cancer choice, especially if you feel uncertain about making a decision. Firmly ask each specialist you consult to report his findings back to you and your family doctor. This way your family doctor will be in an excellent position to help you sort through and choose an option. Also, if you receive treatment from more than one doctor, it's helpful for your family doctor to be able to monitor all treatments for possible interactions or complications.

For older men with a stage A or B tumor, a low Gleason score, a low PSA, and a relatively short life expectancy, watchful waiting may be the ideal choice. However, if you are in relatively good health with the prospect of quite a few good years ahead of you, radical prostatectomy or radiation therapy will probably be your best bet.

Because of study differences, it's difficult to compare surgery with radiation. At the 10-year mark, there seem to be no major differences between the two treatments. Whether differences develop after 10 years or more is not certain.

Cryosurgery is also a treatment option, although it is still considered experimental. If freezing your prostate cancer cells seems to be the best choice for you, be sure you have the procedure performed at a medical school or institution that is actively studying and attempting to improve this operation.

It may help in making a choice if you take a close look at the pros and cons and risks of side effects for each treatment outlined in this chapter. Some men choose a treatment based on how well they think they will be able to cope with possible side effects.

Meanwhile, the best way to treat prostate cancer remains a matter of debate. Although long-term studies are underway that hope to provide clear answers to this perplexing problem, results won't be available for another 10 years.

Finally, remember that although you can use the stage and grade of your cancer as a general guide in choosing a treatment, you must take your needs and preferences into consideration. It's also important to keep yourself up-to-date on what's happening in the prostate cancer research world. With researchers working worldwide to discover the most effective treatment, one hopes that day won't be far off.

*The natural force within each one of us
is the greatest healer of disease.*
Hippocrates, an ancient Greek physician
commonly considered the Father of Medicine

10

Set your natural healing forces in motion

Battle plan for winning the war against cancer

Part of the reason cancer occurs is that your immune system becomes overwhelmed. It is no longer able to efficiently protect you from dangerous cancer-causing cells, and you develop a full blown case of this deadly disease.

Disheartening as this may sound, knowing this fact can actually help you bring your immune system back up to par so it will fight off those nasty cancer cells. While your doctors will do all they can medically to destroy the mutant cells, you must get your immune system into high gear for their efforts to pay off.

This means keeping your mind, body, and spirit in balance as well as giving your body the best nourishment you can. Just keep in mind that these aspects of healing should always be used in combination with traditional treatments and not in place of them.

2 tips to put you on the right track

It's a frightening experience to hear your doctor say, "You have cancer." However, it's no longer a death sentence as it often was years ago. Today, with new treatments and greater knowledge, it's a whole new ballgame. Along with your medical treatments, here are some self-help strategies that can give you a better crack at recovery.

Practice positive thinking. Study after study shows that attitude affects health. If you have cancer, your attitude has a big influence on your condition.

In a study at UCLA, researchers found that people with cancer live longer when they are relaxed and optimistic about their chances of survival. A six-week program of relaxation techniques, coping strategies, and cancer education resulted in a higher percentage of long-term survival for a group of people with deadly skin cancer. Another group the same age, sex, and with the same seriousness of cancer didn't receive counseling, and their survival rate was one-fifth lower.

For more suggestions on ways to keep your body, mind, and spirit in balance, look for Greg Anderson's inspiring book, *50 Essential Things to Do When the Doctor Says It's Cancer*. A cancer survivor himself, Anderson clearly explains what it takes to live with and overcome cancer.

Join a group. Doctors at universities in New York and California found that people with cancer live longer, happier lives when they join support groups. This proved true for groups of women with breast cancer as well as for groups of men with prostate cancer. Talking with others who have the same disease, and lending each other psychological and emotional support, helps restore self-esteem and confidence. It also reduces depression.

For a list of support groups for prostate cancer, see Chapter 15.

Gear up your immune system

In any battle, the best defense is a prepared defense. This is especially true when it comes to defending your body against

---

Toss the tobacco

If you really want to defeat prostate cancer, stop using all tobacco products. They increase your risk of dying from this disease. Toss 'em all out so you won't even be tempted.

prostate cancer. There are a number of things you can do to help your immune system beat back a cancer attack.

Go for the veggies, fruits, and grains. These foods are high in cancer-fighting antioxidants as well as important vitamins and minerals that can help your immune system mount its strongest defense.

Vanquish with vitamins. Researchers know that ample vitamin D can help prevent prostate cancer. Amazingly enough, new research suggests vitamin D may even be able to slow the growth of prostate cancer.

Studies show that men with prostate cancer often have low levels of vitamin D in their bodies. Since sunlight helps your body produce vitamin D, and vitamin D seems to slow prostate tumor growth, be sure you spend at least 30 minutes in the sun every day.

Other vitamins that may help bolster your immune system include zinc, vitamin B6 (improves the absorption of zinc), selenium, beta carotene, and vitamins C and E. A balanced diet and a good multivitamin will give you a good start on all these nutrients.

A current study at the Medical College of Pennsylvania and Hahnemann University is attempting to determine if a strict low-fat diet and megadoses of vitamins will slow the progression of prostate cancer. Besides eating the low-fat diet, each participant takes 25,000 to 150,000 I.U. of vitamin A, 1,000 to 3,000 I.U. of vitamin E, and 1,000 I.U. of vitamin D. Perhaps their results will offer new hope to men with prostate cancer.

If you wish to try additional supplementation, consult a professional nutritionist who has experience in caring for people with cancer. Also, make sure your doctor knows and OK's any additional supplements you take.

Wash it all down with lots of water. You may not think of water as a nutrient you need, but actually it's one of the few you simply can't do without. If you don't get enough water, any other nutrients you take in will be left high and dry.

A lack of water also interferes with the proper functioning of your immune system, so it's important to make sure you're drinking enough. Drink at least eight 8-ounce glasses of water a day. If your urine is clear or pale yellow, you'll know you're getting enough.

Top it off with the essential "E." Talk about an essential "E," and most people immediately think vitamin E. However, in this case, exercise is just as essential to beating cancer as any vitamin.

Like many of the other things discussed in this chapter, exercise boosts your immune system. Exercise stimulates white blood cells in your immune system called macrophages. These cells are your first line of defense against invaders like viruses, bacteria, and cancer.

Because exercise slightly damages soft tissue, macrophages are routinely called upon to repair the tissue. According to researchers, this may keep them in shape for fighting tumor cells.

Your general goal is to exercise until you feel an increase in energy. This may be as little as five minutes or less of walking at first, especially if you are out of shape or have been weakened by cancer treatments.

Be sure to get the OK from your doctor before you begin. And remember that "E" for exercise also includes the "E" in enjoyment so try to engage in exercise you enjoy. This will make it easier to stick with a regular program.

Say yes to the super healer. Sleep is essential for helping your body recover from illness or injury. It also bolsters your immune system for the needs of tomorrow. In sleep, your body replenishes the cells needed to fend off infections and diseases. One study showed that losing just one night of sleep lowers the action of tumor-fighting blood cells by as much as 30 percent.

Make sure you get at least eight hours of sleep every night. You will probably need more while you're undergoing treatments. Don't deprive yourself of this rest — your body needs it to heal.

The right foods pack a powerful punch

Recently, researchers from the famed Memorial Sloan-Kettering Cancer Center in New York noted that environmental, dietary, and metabolic factors all appear to play a part in prostate cancer's progression. More interestingly, they commented that using traditional cancer therapies as well as modifying the diet "may be appropriate at each stage of cancer growth."

Numerous earlier studies provide support for the position of these researchers. Study after study shows that eating the right foods can make a real difference in whether prostate cancer progresses or not. Based on what many studies have found, here's what experts suggest:

Live low-fat. Researchers at Memorial Sloan-Kettering Cancer Center have found that a low-fat diet seems to slow the growth of prostate cancer. Human prostate tumors injected into mice grew only half as fast in mice who ate diets with 21 percent fat compared to those who ate 40 percent fat.

Some dietary fats are more dangerous than others. The most harmful fats are contained in meats, eggs, cheese, cream, hydrogenated vegetable oils, butter, mayonnaise, salad dressings, and many baked goods.

Poultry fat, on the other hand, has not been linked to prostate cancer. And Omega-3 fatty acids from fish oils seem to suppress tumor growth.

Limit meat. In countries where people eat a lot of meat and fats, there are many more cases of prostate cancer than in other countries. In a Harvard University study, men who ate beef, lamb, and pork nearly every day suffered from worse complications of prostate cancer 2-1/2 times more often than men who ate meat as little as once a month. A low-fat, high-fiber diet reduces the risk that microscopic cancers will spread and become life-threatening.

Get plenty of protein. Although you want to limit meat, you still need to be sure you have enough protein in your diet. Protein provides energy, helps you maintain your strength, and rebuilds tissues that may have been affected by your cancer treatments. Other good sources of protein besides meat include nonfat dairy foods, soy products, legumes, seeds, and nuts.

Fill up on fiber. Enjoy whole-grain breads and at least five servings of fruits and vegetables every day. High-fiber vegetables include broccoli, cabbage, brussels sprouts, and legumes, such as dried beans, lentils, peas, and lima beans. Eat fresh vegetables raw, steamed, or microwaved.

Fresh or dried fruits, such as raisins and dates, are also good sources of fiber. For the best benefits, leave the skins on fresh fruits.

Favor fresh. Choose fresh over canned or frozen foods whenever possible. Fresh foods generally offer more bang for your nutritional buck than canned, frozen, boxed, or bottled foods.

Bring on the soy. Soy products are a rich source of chemical agents that suppress tumor growth. More than 100 studies have demonstrated that genistein, one of the compounds in soy that has recently received a lot of attention, can actually stop the growth of cancer cells.

Researchers believe genistein can curb the growth of prostate cancer in three different ways. First, it appears to block those enzymes in the body responsible for converting normal cells to cancer cells. Second, genistein appears to interfere with the hormones that prostate cancers need to grow. Third, it seems genistein may also interfere with the tumor's process of receiving nutrients and oxygen, which it also must have to grow.

Although more research must be done to determine how to best use genistein to help men with prostate cancer or to determine if eating soy can help inhibit tumor growth, it certainly won't harm you (and may even help) if you eat tofu or other soy products on a daily basis.

It's really quite easy to work into your regular meals. For example, you can substitute soy for meat in lasagna, chili, or stir-fry recipes. Soft tofu is good in salad dressings, dips, and milkshakes. You can make a half-and-half mixture of soy milk and regular milk for your breakfast cereal, pudding, cream soups, and sauces. Try adding miso (another soy food) to soup, or grill sliced tempeh and vegetables for a healthy soy meal.

Kick caffeine and alcohol habits. These drinks tend to deplete your body of needed nutrients. Also, avoid refined sugar and white flour because they have little nutritional value.

For more information on eating nutritionally while battling cancer, check out the following publications:

A Guide to Good Nutrition During and After Chemotherapy and Radiation, by S. Aker, 1988. This publication includes specific food suggestions, plus recipes, charts, and a calorie and protein guide. To order, call (206) 467-4834.

Eating Hints for Cancer Patients, 1995. This 94-page booklet includes information on dietary needs, suggested menus, and recipes. To order, call 1-800-4-CANCER (1-800-422-6237).

Pectin power to the rescue

Although many prostate cancers don't spread, or are caught and cured before spreading, some still manage to slip out into the bloodstream or lymph system. Those that do metastasize usually aren't curable.

While some natural therapies, such as a low-fat diet and plenty of vitamin D, may slow the progression of prostate cancer, only genistein (a component of soy products) has been able to completely stop the spread of prostate cancer — until now, that is.

Preliminary research on mice suggests that pieces of pectin (a popular ingredient used in canning jams and jellies) may also be able to put the spread of prostate cancer on hold, perhaps permanently.

In a study conducted at Wayne State University in Detroit, researchers found that rats injected with prostate cancer who drank water supplemented with the researchers' special version of pectin developed less than half as many metastases as rats drinking plain water.

The researchers think the pectin works by preventing tumor cells from attaching themselves to blood vessel walls. Without the blood vessels to nourish them, the cancer cells can't spread. Although the main research was done with prostate cancer, researchers think their results would apply to almost any other cancer — good news for everyone fighting this difficult battle.

Since the research is still in its early stages, pectin is not yet available for widespread use. And while pectin is a natural product found on grocery store shelves everywhere, the researchers caution against trying to medicate yourself with pectin. It won't help since the researchers have to put the pectin through a special process that allows it to be absorbed by the body.

Taking pure pectin off the shelf is just like eating dietary fiber or drinking Metamucil. You may be more "regular," but it won't give a strategic advance in winning your war against prostate cancer.

Natural healer offers new hope

When it comes to promoting good health, garlic is one of Mother Nature's most powerful healers. From major problems like heart disease to minor irritations like swimmer's ear, garlic both protects and heals your body. In fact, garlic has been used both as food and medicine since the earliest Chinese dynasties.

Now, new test-tube experiments from Memorial Sloan-Kettering Cancer Center suggest aged garlic may even be able to slow the progression of prostate cancer.

Researchers took a substance found in aged garlic called S-allylmercaptocysteine (SAMC) and applied it to live cells very similar to prostate cancer cells. SAMC was able to slow the cancer

Can prostate cancer be reversed?

Once again Dr. Dean Ornish is out to do the undoable.

World-renowned for his landmark studies on how lifestyle changes could reverse heart disease, he's now out to prove that lifestyle changes may be able to stop or reverse prostate cancer.

In an ongoing study of 100 men in the San Francisco Bay area, Ornish is testing whether stress reduction and an extremely low-fat diet can put a stop to prostate cancer. Men under Ornish's plan will consume only 10 percent of their calories from fat. On average, most American diets consist of 40 percent fat.

Ornish's interest in trying his plan on men with prostate cancer was sparked by a study conducted by William Fair, M.D., chief of urology at Memorial Sloan-Kettering Hospital in New York. Dr. Fair's study found that prostate cancer growth was halted in mice whose fat consumption was limited to around 20 percent.

cells' growth by about 70 percent. The garlic also decreased the amounts of two other proteins in the body that tend to promote prostate cancer.

The concentrations researchers used to slow the cancer's growth would be similar to those levels that could develop in the blood of people taking commercially aged garlic pills. However, you won't get the same benefits the researchers saw in the study by flavoring your foods with fresh garlic. The garlic needs to have been aged for at least a year.

It is not yet clear whether the effect the aged garlic had on cancer cells in the lab will translate into any benefit for humans eating aged garlic. More studies are underway that hope to find out.

Wonder cure is more hype than help

Despite all the hype and positive press about shark cartilage preventing cancer, the latest research concludes it's more likely to shrink your wallet than your tumor.

One of the most recent studies of shark cartilage followed 60 people with advanced cancers (mainly of the breast, colon, lung, and prostate) for 10 months. None of the participants was taking standard anti-cancer drugs.

Each participant took large amounts of powdered shark cartilage dissolved in juice or flavored water three times a day. To get that same amount in capsules, the subjects would have had to take 100 or more 500-milligram capsules a day. That much shark cartilage would cost the average person about $1,000 per month.

Since sharks rarely get cancer, researchers had originally theorized that some substance in sharks' cartilage may protect against the disease by slowing the growth of blood vessels needed for tumor development.

Unfortunately, none of the participants showed any signs of either partial or total remission of their cancer. However, some natural healers still feel shark cartilage can be a useful addition to traditional treatments and diet changes. Other studies examining shark cartilage's effect on cancer are ongoing.

If you're determined to take shark cartilage, the good news is it probably won't hurt you, although you should check with your doctor before you begin supplements. However, you also can't be sure it won't interfere with your other treatments. Besides being expensive and unhelpful, side effects of shark cartilage may include nausea and vomiting.

In summary

The key to controlling cancer is bolstering your immune system. This means keeping your mind, body, and spirit in balance as well as giving your body the very best nourishment you can.

Maintaining a positive attitude has an important impact on your health. Also, be sure to link up with others who have prostate cancer. This is a good way for you to both give and receive emotional support.

Nutritionwise, your best bet for beating cancer is to focus on a food plan that emphasizes vegetables, fruits, and grains. It's also important to make sure you're getting all the vitamins you need. Many people with cancer find it helpful to consult a qualified nutritionist.

Now is the time to break all those bad habits you've been harboring over the years. Toss your tobacco products, and just say no to alcohol and caffeine. While tobacco actually increases your risk of dying from cancer, alcohol and caffeine deplete your body of nutrients your immune system needs to fight the disease.

Other quick and easy ways to give your overworked immune system an easy boost include drinking eight 8-ounce glasses of water every day, exercising regularly, and getting at least eight hours of sleep every night.

Along with good medical treatment, taking care of yourself is the best way to take cancer out of the game.

Your heaviest artillery will be your will to live.
Keep that big gun going.
Norman Cousins, author of *Anatomy of an Illness.*
His own near escape from a life-threatening condition
led him to explore the powerful effect
a positive attitude can have on serious illness.

11

Advanced prostate cancer

Unfortunately, no cure for advanced prostate cancer yet exists. However, new developments that may offer the possibility of cure include a prostate cancer vaccine, which shows signs of being able to reverse even advanced cancer, and a specially engineered killer virus. Significant advances in gene therapy also look promising.

Options that help you live a longer, better life

While researchers work on perfecting treatments that offer new hope to men with advanced prostate cancer, you have some options already available that can help you live a longer, more fulfilling life right now. In addition, you may find it encouraging to note that prostate cancer survival rates are much higher (more than three times as high in many cases) than most other forms of cancer. On average, the five-year survival rate for advanced prostate cancer is 28 percent.

Generally, the first goal of your urologist will be to slow the progression of advanced prostate cancer. Next, he'll work with you to deal with the bone pain and general feelings of discomfort many men with advanced prostate cancer experience. Older men with other significant health problems or a shorter estimated lifespan sometimes choose more conservative treatments to spare themselves unpleasant side effects of treatment.

Hormone therapy throws a one-two punch

Since the 1940s, most doctors' strategic defense for slowing the progression of advanced prostate cancer has been to cut off the supply of androgens. Because most prostate cancers need the hormone testosterone (a type of androgen) to fuel their growth, this technique usually produces a reliable, if not a dramatic, response.

This is where hormone therapy comes in. Using two different approaches, either surgery or drugs, you can stop or significantly slow the production of testosterone or interfere with its effect on the prostate. This usually helps slow the cancer's growth as well as relieve pain. Knowing some basic facts about how hormones are produced in the body can help you understand how this process works.

An area in your brain called the hypothalamus gives the signal to start testosterone production. It does this by secreting luteinizing hormone-releasing hormone (LHRH) at regular intervals. In turn, LHRH prompts your pituitary gland (also located in the brain) to produce luteinizing hormone (LH). Finally, LH tells the Leydig cells in your prostate to release testosterone into your bloodstream. Once testosterone reaches the prostate, the enzyme called 5-alpha reductase converts it to a more potent form of testosterone — dihydrotestosterone (DHT).

Surgery cuts this process off at the testicles. With the testicles gone, they can no longer receive signals from the brain to produce testosterone. Drugs, depending on what type they are, interfere with this process at several different stages.

Although hormone therapy can sometimes control cancer that has spread beyond the prostate, it isn't a cure. However, this treatment usually helps about 80 to 85 percent of men with advanced prostate cancer. Most men will continue to respond to hormone treatment for one-and-a-half to four years.

Other benefits may include tumor shrinkage, relief of urinary problems, less bone pain, better appetite, and milder anemia. Hormone therapy may be used alone or in combination with surgery or radiation therapy.

The benefits stop when hormone therapy is stopped. Also, side effects may put a damper on your sex life as they generally include impotence and a loss of interest in sex. However, hormone therapy won't decrease your interest in aspects of intimacy, such as hugs and kisses. Also, you can still engage in sexual experiences that don't require an erection. If sex is still a very important part of your life, you may want to keep these things in mind when making a choice about hormone therapy. Many men also experience hot flashes and weight gain.

In addition, how well hormone therapy works for you depends on how sensitive your cancer cells are to hormones. The more hormone-sensitive your cancer cells are, the better you will do on this type of therapy. If your PSA levels fall to 4 ng/mL or less during the first six months, this suggests you will probably respond well to hormone therapy.

You may want to keep in mind that the timing of hormone therapy doesn't appear to affect survival. In fact, one study found that survival rates were the same for men who started hormone therapy early as they were for men who started hormone therapy later. However, some doctors believe that hormone therapy does slow prostate cancer's progression, and they like to begin hormone therapy as soon as it's clear the prostate cancer has metastasized. This, of course, usually means impotence and a general lack of interest in sex.

Other doctors see no point in subjecting men to the sexual side effects when it's not clear that early hormone treatment can increase survival. They prefer to postpone hormone therapy until the prostate cancer begins causing symptoms, such as urinary difficulty or pain.

However, most doctors will recommend that you begin hormone therapy immediately if you have pain, urinary difficulties, anemia, weight loss, swelling, shortness of breath, or show signs that the cancer may be affecting your nervous system.

Types of hormone therapy

Orchiectomy. Removing the testicles, the factories that produce 90 to 95 percent of the body's testosterone, is a time-tested way to effectively stop testosterone production and slow the cancer's spread. Although orchiectomy is technically a type of surgery, it's generally grouped under hormone therapy because the point of the procedure is to shut off your body's supply of the hormone testosterone.

If you choose this option, you will have a bilateral orchiecto-my (removal of both testicles). During the 20-minute operation, which generally only requires local anesthesia, the testicles alone are removed. Everything else, such as the scrotum and the penis, are left in place. Prosthetic testicles are available that make it look as if the testes are still present.

About three hours after surgery, testosterone levels will drop by 95 percent. This is called the castrate range. The effectiveness of hormone drugs is determined by how they compare to the castrate range produced by surgery.

Although many men fear that this procedure brings any sort of sex life to a premature end, that is not necessarily the case. After surgery, some men keep their sexual desires and abilities for a long time. However, the testicles are the manufacturing plant of testosterone, which plays a big role in sex drive. The shutting down of the plant does eventually put many men out of the sex business.

If you have an orchiectomy, you'll need to lavish some extra loving attention on your bones. According to a recent study, men who have one or both testicles removed are at greater risk from suffering a broken bone as the result of osteoporosis (a bone-thinning disease that often affects women). To reduce this risk, make sure you walk regularly or get other exercise, and take 1,500 mg of calcium a day to maintain your bone strength.

Pros

▶ Most effective and least expensive way to shut down testosterone production.

▶ A safe, one-time treatment. No need for a lifetime of medication or monthly shots.

Cons

▶ Removal of testicles is irreversible.

▶ Appears to cause a higher risk of osteoporosis-related bone fractures.

▶ The psychological side effects of this treatment are severe for some men.

Estrogen. Estrogen stops testosterone from being produced by the testicles by blocking the release of LH from the pituitary gland. Usually doctors prescribe diethylstilbestrol, also known as DES.

Although estrogen is not an expensive method of treating advanced cancer, it is not often used because it can cause serious side effects in men with a history of heart disease or blood clots.

Pros

▶ Fairly cheap.

▶ Treatment is reversible.

Cons

▶ May cause serious side effects in men with heart disease or a history of blood clots.

▶ May stimulate breast growth, which will also be irreversible. However, undergoing radiation treatment before taking estrogen may prevent breast growth.

Luteinizing hormone-releasing hormone (LHRH) agonists. The most commonly used hormone therapy for prostate cancer, LHRH agonists also shut off the supply of testosterone from the testicles by blocking the pituitary's production of LH. Treatment is often supplied in the form of monthly injections. A longer-lasting version that you receive every three months is also available now.

At the beginning of LHRH agonist treatment, there is often an increase in LHRH, which causes more testosterone to be produced. This may cause you to have what's called a flare reaction, in which tumor-related symptoms, such as bone pain, urinary problems, and even spinal cord compression, temporarily worsen. If your cancer has spread to the bone, doctors normally block this effect by giving you an antiandrogen for two weeks before you receive the LHRH agonist shot.

Commonly used LHRH agonists include leuprolide acetate (Lupron) and goserelin acetate (Zoladex).

Pros

▶ Generally causes fewer side effects than estrogen.

▶ Treatment is reversible.

Cons

▶ One of the more expensive forms of hormone therapy.

▶ Must go to doctor's office every one to three months to receive the shot.

Antiandrogens. These drugs interfere with testosterone's ability to bind with androgen receptors in the prostate gland's cells. If they can't bind, the cancer can't grow. Antiandrogens also block testosterone from the adrenal glands, small glands that sit on top of the kidneys and produce only 5 to 10 percent of your body's testosterone. Unfortunately,. antiandrogens used by themselves aren't very effective.

Antiandrogens are often combined with LHRH agonists to block testosterone produced both by the adrenal glands and the testicles. This type of combination therapy is often referred to as a total androgen blockade or combined androgen deprivation.

Some commonly used antiandrogens include bicalutamide (Casodex), finasteride (Proscar), and flutamide (Eulexin). Although flutamide is still generally considered safe, researchers have noted a higher-than-expected rate of liver damage in men using this drug. To prevent this problem, men using flutamide need to have their liver function tested within a few months of beginning treatment.

Pros

▶ Treatment is reversible.

Cons

▶ Pills, especially if used to create a total androgen blockage, must be taken several times a day.

▶ Expensive.

See Chapter 16 for more information on the different drugs discussed in this chapter.

Combination hormone therapy. Recently the National Cancer Institute completed a study of combination hormone therapy that paired a nonsteroidal antiandrogen and a luteinizing hormone-releasing hormone agonist. Results were promising. Combining the antiandrogen flutamide and the LHRH agonist leuprolide increased survival time by 25 percent. On average, the men taking the combination lived 35.6 months, which is 7.3 months longer than survival time for men taking leuprolide alone.

Even better, the combination also slowed the cancer's progression. On average, for men on the combination treatment, 16.5 months passed before the cancer progressed compared to 13.9 months for men taking only leuprolide.

However, other recent studies question the real benefits of long-term combination hormone therapy or a total androgen blockade. If you're interested in trying combination treatment or a total androgen blockade but you're confused by the controversy, ask your doctor to keep you posted on the latest findings.

You can also keep yourself up to date if you have access to a medical library. In addition, the Internet is a good source of late-breaking information on controversial treatments. See Chapter 2 for more tips on navigating the Internet.

Radiation to resist cancer pain

Radiotherapy is another good option for relieving bone pain. Normally, up to 10 sessions of radiation will provide effective pain relief. Sometimes, doctors will also recommend radiation before pain becomes noticeable, particularly in areas prone to pain, such as the spine and thighs. Preventive radiation can also lessen the likelihood that fractures will occur.

Recently, a study was done of 401 men aged 51 to 80 with locally advanced cancer. Those who underwent seven weeks of radiation along with an injection of goserelin (Zoladex) every four weeks had improved control of the cancer. They also lived longer. Five-year survival rates were 79 percent for the men in the combined treatment group compared with a 62 percent survival rate in the men who received radiation only.

Research takes its best shot against cancer

Smallpox was once a major killer, claiming the lives of millions. Then Edward Jenner discovered a vaccine that was so effective that the world was declared officially smallpox-free in 1979. Now researchers are busy working on a vaccine for today's number one killer — cancer. Prostate cancer may be the most likely candidate for the first successful cancer vaccine.

Most vaccines contain weakened or "killed" versions of the germ that causes the disease they are designed to prevent. The vaccine is then injected into a person, which stimulates the immune system to attack the germs. Once you receive a vaccine, you are protected from the disease because your immune system recognizes that specific germ and knows to attack it quickly, before it has time to harm your body.

One of the reasons prostate cancer is so common is that your immune system often doesn't recognize an excess of PSA as a warning signal of cancer, so it doesn't properly defend your body. However, one researcher, Dr. Gerald Murphy, has had some early success with a new prostate vaccine. Unlike most vaccines, which are given before you get the disease, this promising new treatment is for men who already have prostate cancer.

Murphy and his colleagues studied 57 volunteers with advanced prostate cancer that had not responded to conventional treatment. They were only trying to show that their treatment was safe. Unexpectedly, however, seven of the men showed improvement. One man, whose cancer had metastasized to his bones, experienced dramatic improvement. His PSA level fell to an undetectable level, he gained weight, his bones showed no more signs of cancer, and he became pain-free.

The vaccine is made from the blood of men with advanced prostate cancer. Researchers take immune system cells called dendritic cells, grow them in a laboratory, and combine them with prostate specific membrane antigens. They then inject this solution into the bloodstream, and it travels to different areas of the body, such as the lymph nodes and spleen. There, it attracts cancer-killing T-cells, which learn to seek out and attack other cells containing PSA.

Although this treatment is still in the experimental stages, more studies are underway now, and it could lead to more effective treatments, not just for prostate cancer, but for all cancers.

Ingenious prostate protection

You get a lot from genes. You may have gotten the genes for your crystal blue eyes from your mother, and the genes for your irresistible charm from your father. However, interesting new research suggests genes may give you more than good looks, a sparkling personality, or your lightning-fast brain. Now, scientists think genes may provide special substances that protect you from prostate cancer.

Researchers are working on techniques for gene therapy to help control prostate cancer. One method being investigated at UCLA's Jonsson Comprehensive Cancer Center involves synthetically created genes.

The gene produces a substance called interleukin-2 (IL-2) that attracts "killer cells" or lymphocytes from your immune system. Doctors inject the gene directly into your prostate, and your lymphocytes move in for the kill. After a while, the cancer cells start to produce IL-2 on their own, helping your lymphocytes to recognize them as dangerous. They will then be able to track down prostate cancer cells that may have migrated to other parts of your body. Prostate cancer cells are particularly partial to bone.

Another similar technique being studied involves genetically engineering prostate cancer cells to express a substance called B7, which causes T-cells from your immune system to attack. Then the T-cells will attack other prostate cells, even if they don't produce B7.

These new techniques provide an advantage over traditional cancer treatments because they can fight cancerous cells throughout your body. And they do it without causing harm to healthy tissue, like chemotherapy can.

Although gene therapy also is still in experimental stages, it remains one of the bright hopes for the future of cancer treatment.

Your cold may kill your cancer

You've probably spent a lot of time trying to avoid colds. Meanwhile, researchers have spent a lot of time trying to figure out how to cure or prevent them. Although scientists may never find a cure for the common cold, they may have discovered the next best thing — a way to make cold viruses useful.

Researchers at the Johns Hopkins Oncology Center have produced a mutant strain of the common cold virus that attacks and kills only prostate cells. The virus is programmed to be activated by the presence of PSA in a cell. Therefore, although the virus can enter any cell of your body, it only destroys cells with PSA — prostate cells.

The virus attacks healthy prostate cells as well as cancerous ones; but many prostate treatments, such as prostatectomy, also remove healthy prostate tissue.

The virus therapy has only been tested on mice, but the results were promising. According to one report, a single injection shrank tumors to an average of only 16 percent of their original size. Studies on humans are due to begin soon.

Combat complications of advanced cancer

When the cancer spreads to lower vertebrae of your spine, it may cause both urination difficulties and spinal cord compression. The latter is a serious problem that can lead to paralysis.

Undergoing a transurethral resection of the prostate (TURP) can relieve the urination problems. TURP is a commonly used procedure for BPH. For more information on this fairly simple surgery, see Chapter 4.

Treating spinal cord compression is a little more involved. If you haven't already begun hormone therapy, most doctors will probably recommend a bilateral orchiectomy. If you've been taking hormones and your testosterone levels have dropped into the castrate range, most doctors will begin steroids. They also will set up an appointment with a neurosurgeon to determine if you need surgery to relieve the pressure on your spine.

Signs of a possible spinal cord compression may include extreme weakness in your lower body and difficulty in controlling bowel movements. If you have any of these symptoms, let your doctor know immediately. If you can't reach your doctor, go to the nearest emergency room.

When it's time for other treatments

Prostate cancer is made up of both androgen-dependent cells, which need androgen hormones to grow; and androgen-independent cells, which don't need those hormones to grow. Unfortunately, hormone therapy only works on the cells that are hormone-dependent. Meanwhile, their independent brothers continue to multiply until eventually the therapy becomes ineffective.

Recently, doctors have been trying intermittent androgen suppression (using an LHRH agonist alone or with an antiandrogen) to delay the take-over by the deadly hormone-independent cells. Hormone therapy is continued until PSA levels drop. It is resumed only when PSA levels begin to climb again. Although side effects are reduced with this treatment, researchers aren't sure about the effectiveness of this approach. Studies are underway to evaluate the effects on survival time.

For many men, hormone therapy only works for one-and-a-half to four years before it becomes ineffective. When that happens, it's time to consider other treatment options.

Chemotherapy

When prostate cancer has progressed to the point that it no longer needs androgens to grow, hormone therapy will no longer be helpful. At this point, you and your doctor may decide it's time to try chemotherapy.

Traditionally, chemotherapy works by using very powerful drugs that slow the rate of cell growth in the body. Although these drugs harm both the healthy and the cancerous cells in your body, they usually target cells growing the fastest — typically cancer cells and hair cells, which explains the hair loss many people on chemotherapy experience. Other side effects may include nausea, tiredness, and general body pain.

Although chemotherapy hasn't proven that useful in the past for slowing prostate cancer, new developments may have more to offer. Part of the problem with past chemotherapy attempts to control prostate cancer is that chemotherapy drugs generally target cells that are dividing much faster than prostate cancer cells.

Newer drugs that target growth factors look more promising. One such drug, called suramin, offers new hope because it may work on hormone-resistant cells. Side effects may include skin rash, longer periods of bleeding, and disorders of the cornea (the front part of the eyeball).

Another promising chemotherapy drug recently approved by the FDA is called mitoxantrone (Novantrone). Combined with corticosteriods, this drug is helpful for those men who are no longer responsive to hormone therapy. The drug also lowers PSA levels, which offers many men peace of mind in addition to relief from pain. (Rising PSA levels often suggest the cancer is progressing.) Side effects may include nausea, fatigue, hair loss, appetite loss, constipation, and breathing difficulty. A small number of men taking the drug experience heart complications.

Yet another promising option is estramustine phosphate sodium (Emcyt), which has been reported to help between 30 and 60 percent of the men who try it. As with all chemotherapeutic drugs, side effects can be severe, especially in older men who are somewhat frail.

More methods of pain relief

Other options for pain relief include drugs called biophosphonates and injections of strontium-89 (a radioactive substance used to relieve the pain of cancer that has spread to the bones). Nonsteroidal anti-inflammatory drugs (NSAIDs), corticosteroids, and morphine or other narcotics can also offer effective pain relief.

If pain becomes suddenly intense or extremely severe, doctors sometimes suggest ketoconazole, a drug typically used to treat fungal infections. However, it also stops the production of androgens produced by the testicles and adrenal glands. It will reduce testosterone levels within 24 hours, so it's a fairly quick method of pain relief. However, it's not recommended for long-term relief as it may eventually cause testosterone levels to rise again. Also, it may damage your liver.

Sometimes you may be able to try experimental drugs that have not yet been approved by the FDA by participating in a clinical trial. See Chapter 9 for more information on clinical trials, and ask your doctor if he knows of any trials you may be eligible to participate in.

If you think you need a higher dose or a different medicine for pain relief, don't hesitate to ask your doctor, and be firm about your request. While it's your job to let your doctor know about whatever pain you have, it's his job to help you get the pain relief you need.

Why you need a durable power of attorney

If you become so sick that you are not able to make decisions, you'll need someone to make decisions for you. However, it's not as simple as saying to your wife or children who you want to be in charge of your health care decisions. You have to legally designate the person you've chosen, or your family or friend won't be able to make any decisions for you without going through a long and costly legal process.

The easiest way to solve this problem is to set up a durable power of attorney for health care and/or financial decisions. When you set up a durable power of attorney, you appoint a trusted relative or friend to make business, property, asset, financial, and health decisions for you when you can't.

You give that person the right to handle financial matters that include paying bills, making bank deposits, dealing with insurance, and selling a home or other property. Your agent may also use your funds to pay for your medical expenses that aren't covered by Medicare or health insurance. The more specific your instructions, the better your agent will handle your affairs and your health care decisions.

Protect your health care with a living will

Thanks to a 1990 decision by the United States Supreme Court, you are entitled to direct your own medical care — not only while you're healthy but after you're incapacitated, too.

Most states have a form containing specific language that you use to spell out the type of medical treatment you want to receive if you have a terminal illness or become comatose. It's called a living will, a health care advance directive, or a directive to physicians. The medical staff must follow your directions exactly. Neither family wishes nor doctor beliefs can override your directives in states that recognize them.

Laws concerning living wills vary from state to state, particularly concerning formalities like witnesses and notarization. You can obtain specific information on your state's laws, and the forms to fill out, from:

Legal Counsel for the Elderly (LCE)
American Association of Retired Persons
P.O. Box 96474
Washington, D.C. 20090-6474

You simply fill out the preprinted form. The format of these forms also varies from state to state, but for every form, you'll need to consider such issues as:

- If breathing is labored or ceases, do you want to be kept alive with a ventilator or respirator?

- If you are unable to eat, do you want a feeding tube or intravenous line inserted, or do you want food and water withheld? What about other life-sustaining treatment?

- Do you want pain relievers, and if so, how often?

Give a copy of your living will to your doctor and to the family member most likely to be responsible for your care should you become unable. Also, make sure a copy is on file at the hospital where you will most likely be treated.

Overcoming cancer

At this point, overcoming cancer is just as much a matter of living your life the way you want to as it is a matter of making it last longer. Those who overcome take their cancer diagnosis as a wake-up call, a reminder that every day is to be lived to the fullest doing the things they love with the ones they love. If you make that your approach, you too have overcome cancer — no matter what the outcome.

In summary

While there is currently no cure for advanced prostate cancer, you do have a number of options for both slowing its progression and preventing pain. Most of these options center around different forms of hormone therapy. By cutting or drastically reducing the supply of androgens (male hormones, especially testosterone), you can often dramatically slow the progression of prostate cancer.

When choosing a method of pain relief, remember to keep your own needs and preferences in mind. Don't be embarrassed or shy about asking questions and telling your doctor what you want. It's your right to demand that everything possible be done both to prolong your life and ease your pain.

Also, be sure to keep abreast of new developments in the treatment of prostate cancer. A prostate cancer vaccine under study shows signs of being able to reverse even advanced prostate cancer.

Finally, remember that no matter what statistics say about how long you're likely to live, you're an individual with an individual destiny. If you refuse to be sucked into the vortex of negative thinking, you may far outlive any statistic. If you take control of the things in your life that you can, the rest of life will take care of itself. It may even turn out better than you expected.

Life consists not in holding good cards
but in playing those you hold well.
Josh Billings, 19th-century American humorist

12

The indignity
of incontinence

Did you know that two out of 10 people can't remember when they last went to the bathroom? If you suffer from incontinence, you may spend so much time in the bathroom you wish you could forget. There may be some comfort in knowing incontinence is a common condition, affecting more than 10 million Americans. But if you've got prostate problems, then urinary troubles may not be far behind.

In fact, for those men who undergo a radical prostatectomy for prostate cancer, the most disturbing side effect is urinary incontinence. It can disrupt all aspects of your daily life from social activities to sexual relations.

The good news is, with a little work, most men regain urinary control. The best news is, even if you can't regain control, there are effective options for dealing with this problem so you can get on with your life the way you used to.

Know your foe — fight
the 4 kinds of incontinence

If you are suffering from incontinence, it could be due to any of several different reasons. Experts have come up with four basic categories to help you separate the symptoms and causes, but all of them mean something is not working quite right.

▶ **Stress incontinence** is the most common type and the most easily cured. You'll notice when you exercise, lift, laugh, sneeze, or cough, that a small amount of urine leaks out. This usually happens when the muscle that controls urine flow, the bladder sphincter, becomes weak. However, if you've had a prostatectomy, the pelvic floor muscles may not be as strong as they once were, or they could have been damaged during surgery. Muscle exercises can cure many suffering from stress incontinence, but if not, you may need to consider an artificial sphincter.

▶ **Urge incontinence** can be caused by a prostate infection, BPH, prostate cancer, or a prostatectomy. You feel the sudden need to urinate, but can't reach the bathroom in time.

▶ **Overflow incontinence** occurs when an enlarged prostate presses against the urethra, blocking the flow of urine out of your body. Your bladder becomes too full, and small amounts of urine dribble out without control.

▶ **Mixed incontinence** is when you experience a combination of these symptoms. For men with an enlarged prostate, the most common diagnosis is urge incontinence and overflow incontinence.

Answer the right questions to get the right diagnosis

Write down the answers to these questions before you see your doctor. It will help him give you a more accurate diagnosis.
- How long have you been having trouble with urine leakage?
- What kind of trouble are you having holding your urine?
- How often do you urinate unexpectedly?
- When do you urinate unexpectedly?
- What activities cause you to leak?
- Do you wear absorbent pads? How often?
- Do you use other protective devices?

Everything you need to know
about the causes of incontinence

Drugs

If you have an enlarged prostate, you could develop overflow incontinence or urinary retention when taking multisymptom cold capsules. The ingredients to watch out for are:

- alpha agonists

- anticholinergic agents

- nasal decongestants

- nonprescription hypnotic antihistamines

If you suffer from BPH, you might find that calcium channel blockers make your incontinence worse. These drugs affect how well the bladder muscles respond to your body's demands. If the muscles in your bladder don't contract as they should, your bladder won't empty and you end up with overflow incontinence.

Conditions

▶ Most men are incontinent after a radical prostatectomy, at least for a few days. Sphincter damage is the main cause of incontinence after surgery for prostate cancer. As things begin to heal, you should see a vast improvement. However, the healing process can take a long time, even up to a year. After that amount of time, if you are still having trouble controlling your urine, you should go to your doctor for help.

▶ Prostatitis may be the reason you are waking in the middle of the night with an urgent need to go to the bathroom. Get help for this because the pattern of waking and urinating results in a large number of fall-related injuries.

▶ Benign prostatic hyperplasia (BPH) can block the urethra and cause urine retention. Drug therapy or surgery are usually prescribed.

▶ Stones in your prostate or bladder can cause the bladder to become infected or swell and no longer function properly.

▶ Chemotherapy for prostate cancer can cause a bladder infection, which in turn can cause incontinence.

Surgery

If you have had surgery for prostate enlargement or cancer, the muscles controlling urine flow may be weakened or damaged.

What you need to know to beat incontinence

Generally, doctors recommend you choose what they call the "least invasive treatment" first. That means trying the option that will have the fewest negative side effects. Usually those are behavior techniques — simple changes you make in your life. However, sometimes taking drugs, using devices, or undergoing surgery are the only way to see improvement. Just discuss all the possible risks, benefits, and outcomes with your doctor.

8 ways to combat incontinence

Here are a few self-care tips to help you manage incontinence due to prostate problems:

Steer clear of alcohol and caffeine. If you're already suffering from incontinence for any reason, alcohol and caffeine should be the first two things you give up. Both of these are diuretics, which mean they increase the amount of urine your body produces.

Beat incontinence with biofeedback. Biofeedback is not something you can start doing all by yourself. You need someone trained in this technique who can walk you through the exercises. They will use an electronic or mechanical device to show you just how your body responds under different situations. Then you will learn how to gradually become more aware of your muscles and how to control them.

Most of the devices record how well you contract your pelvic muscles. This makes the technique especially useful, along with the Kegel exercises. And it can be a very successful program. One study showed biofeedback reduced episodes of incontinence in men who had undergone prostate surgery by up to 80 percent.

If you are willing to find a trained therapist and devote the time needed to make this program work, you could put an end to your incontinence problems.

Learn the benefits of bladder training. This technique teaches you to control your urges and gradually go longer and longer between urinating.

- Go to the toilet every 30 minutes, night and day.

- Very gradually increase the time between your trips until you can go at least two or three hours without an accident. Depending on your control, you may be able to eventually go longer.

This type of therapy improves about 75 percent of the men suffering from urge incontinence.

Change to the diet with a difference. Becoming constipated will only make a bad situation worse. Too much stool impacted near your rectum makes it harder for you to use and control your bladder muscles. So eat plenty of fiber and try to keep regular bowel habits.

Regain control with Kegel exercises. These exercises will strengthen and tone the muscles that control urination. Many doctors recommend you begin these immediately after a radical prostatectomy, but they are useful for other conditions as well.

First, you need to identify which muscles you will be working. One group is actually located around the rectum but is used to stop the flow of urine. The other group of muscles is around the base of the penis. You usually contract these when you are going to the bathroom and trying to get the last amount of urine out. To do the exercises properly, you contract the group near your rectum first, keep those tight, and contract the second group. It may take some concentration the first few times, but you'll soon get the hang of it.

▶ First thing in the morning, urinate in only very small amounts, contracting the muscles in your pelvis every few seconds, at least five times, to stop the stream. Do this until your bladder is empty.

▶ Throughout the day, practice contracting and releasing these muscles even when you're not urinating. Hold them tight for about 10 seconds, relax, and repeat about 15 times. Do this six times a day.

▶ Practice every time you urinate until you can do it easily.

▶ Whenever you are in a situation that normally causes leaking, such as lifting, coughing, etc., consciously tighten these muscles just as you do in practice.

If you're having trouble getting the hang of Kegels, ask your doctor about using biofeedback. Even for men who feel they've mastered Kegels, biofeedback can increase the effectiveness of the exercises. For about six weeks, you'll undergo half-hour training sessions wearing a special undergarment with sensing electrodes. These help you isolate the appropriate muscles and

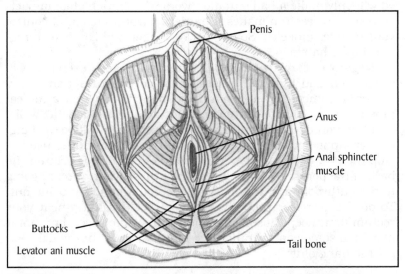

Figure 12.1 - When it comes to regaining your continence, the levator ani muscles are your most important asset. These are the muscles you're contracting when you do your pelvic exercises. Their strength is important because they provide the sling that supports your bladder and other pelvic organs.

improve their strength, which helps immensely in regaining urinary control.

Relax your way to urinary control. If you suffer from urge incontinence and are constantly racing for the bathroom, try these tips to regain a bit of control over this part of your life.

- Relax your stomach muscles.

- Concentrate on waiting.

- Once the urge has passed, go to the bathroom. Walk, don't run. This will help build your physical and mental control.

Timed voiding can turn off incontinence. This plan is especially helpful if you suffer from overflow incontinence. A set schedule keeps your bladder emptied regularly and cuts the risk of involuntary leaking.

▶ Based on how often you find yourself leaking, decide on a voiding schedule. The point is to go to the bathroom before you leak involuntarily. It could be every hour, every two hours, or more.

▶ Empty your bladder completely first thing in the morning, and then begin your schedule for the day.

▶ Try to wait until your next scheduled voiding, even if you feel the need to urinate earlier. Sometimes relaxing or becoming involved in another activity helps.

▶ When your scheduled voiding comes up, try to urinate even if you don't feel the need. This is important since it works the proper muscles.

▶ Record every episode during the day, whether it was a scheduled voiding or an "accident."

Visualize control with visualization. Everyone has used their imagination at least once in their life to get them through a difficult situation. Even though that's a simplified way of explaining visualization, it's one most people can relate to. The real definition is using a picture in your mind to help control body processes.

Many people do this quite easily on their own without any formal training. If you can, that's wonderful. Use it to control your incontinence. For example, if you suffer from urge incontinence picture a dam holding back a river. Or for overflow incontinence, perhaps if you visualize turning off a faucet tighter and tighter, you could squeeze back those annoying dribbles.

But others need guidance, either from a psychotherapist, an alternative learning center, or a book. Through visualization you can learn different ways to soothe, heal, calm, or control your body.

Don't overlook this quick fix

While wearing absorbent pads to protect yourself from embarrassment doesn't really fix your incontinence, there is certainly nothing wrong with it, as long as you're also trying other courses of action. If pads allow you to get on with your life with more confidence, then most experts would encourage you to use them.

There are many new and effective products on the market: pads, shields, guards, bladder control briefs, and adult diapers.

If you choose to use something like this, be sure you take care of your skin. Just as a baby can get diaper rash from wet diapers, you can develop uncomfortable skin irritations from wet pads. To avoid this problem:

- remove the wet article as soon as possible

- clean your skin with warm soapy water

- rinse well

- pat dry

- apply a protective cream or ointment if you choose

Since a rash or irritation here is easily infected, it is extremely important you do all you can to protect your skin.

If your state considers incontinence products to be medical supplies, you don't have to pay sales tax on them. But watch the register. Even if it is a state law, some stores will try to charge tax anyway.

New medical methods to fix the flow

Collagen injections cancel out incontinence. This is a fairly new treatment for men, used to tighten a urethra that is no longer functioning properly after a prostatectomy. It involves injecting collagen, the protein material found in connective tissue, into the area around the urethra. The procedure is done under local anesthesia and has several benefits over older methods. Experts are still concerned, however, over how much the procedure costs and how long the results last.

Make the most of medicines that can mend. If you have stress incontinence, talk to your doctor about taking decongestants. This type of medicine can tighten your bladder muscles and stop involuntary leaking. Don't try this remedy if you suffer from overflow incontinence, however, since it can actually be harmful.

Alpha blockers, the same medicine used to treat high blood pressure, can relieve incontinence symptoms in men with an enlarged prostate. Just be sure your doctor is familiar with your entire medical history before he prescribes these.

Other medicines that your doctor might prescribe for incontinence are:

- propantheline bromide (Pro-Banthine)

- dicyclomine hydrochloride (Bentyl)

- oxybutynin chloride (Ditropan)

- imipramine hydrochloride (Janimine, Tofranil)

- doxepin hydrochloride (Adapin, Sinequan)

- phenylpropanolamine hydrochloride, prolonged release

Not all of these are useful for every type of incontinence, so make sure the prescription fits the cause. See Chapter 16 for more information on these medicines and their possible side effects.

Penile clamps are a prescription for improvement. After prostate surgery, your doctor may advise you to use a penile clamp for a short while. This device squeezes the shaft of the penis so that no urine can flow through. It may sound uncomfortable, but men have been using something like this for many years. It allows them to stay as active as they wish even if they have severe incontinence.

It's very easy to use; you simply remove the clamp about every four hours to go to the bathroom and take it off completely at night. Examine your penis frequently to make sure the clamp is not causing any injury or infection, and don't use it any longer than absolutely necessary. There are plenty of other safer, long-term solutions.

A similar device, the penile cuff, is a comfortable inflatable band that does much the same thing as the penile clamp.

Surgical options provide better control

Weigh the risks of surgery against the possible benefits. Complications such as infection can occur, and in some cases, there are still continence problems after surgery.

Prostate surgery is the best solution for overflow incontinence if it is caused by an enlarged prostate. See Chapters 5 and 6 for more information on surgery for an enlarged prostate.

The artificial sphincter is a three-part device that is surgically implanted near the bladder, in the scrotum, and around the urethra. A cuff keeps the urethra closed until you press the pump in your scrotum. The urethra opens, you are able to urinate, and within a short time, the urethra is forced to close again. Doctors usually suggest you wait at least six months after a prostatectomy before trying this procedure.

The worst way to treat incontinence

Don't try to control your incontinence by decreasing how much you drink. Your body must have a normal amount of fluid every day to keep hydrated.

Many men will stop drinking before an important outing because they don't want any embarrassing accidents. This is foolish since you're quite likely to become dehydrated and could even end up in the hospital.

One estimate claims that between 75 and 85 percent of patients think the artificial sphincter does a satisfactory job. Although not everyone becomes completely continent after the procedure, most are greatly improved. There are some, however, that have problems either with the device itself or with their body's reaction to the surgery. If you decide on this procedure, be aware that you may need a second surgery to either remove or replace the device.

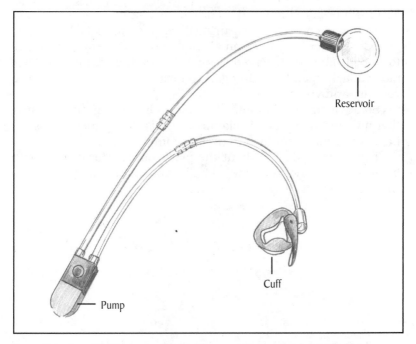

Figure 12.2 - An artificial urinary sphincter. If your continence can't be restored by any other method, the artificial urinary sphincter is an option. Inserted surgically, the pump portion of the artificial sphincter is inserted into the scrotum. The reservoir is placed just under the abdominal muscles. The cuff fits around the urethra just below the external urethral sphincter. The cuff remains inflated until you need to urinate. To urinate, squeeze the scrotum. This activates the pump, which deflates the cuff (sending fluid from the cuff up to the reservoir for temporary storage). This allows urine to flow out of the bladder. The cuff will automatically reinflate in 30 seconds.

In summary

For those men who undergo a radical prostatectomy for prostate cancer, the most disturbing side effect is urinary incontinence. The good news is, with a little work, most men regain urinary control.

Experts have come up with four basic categories of incontinence: stress, urge, overflow, and mixed. They each have their own symptoms and possible remedies.

In addition to prostate surgery, prostatitis, BPH, chemotherapy for prostate cancer, and certain drugs can also cause incontinence.

To regain control of your urine flow, you can make behavioral changes like cutting back on alcohol and caffeine and switching to a high-fiber diet. Or you can learn certain techniques like biofeedback, bladder training, Kegel exercises, relaxation, timed voiding, and visualization.

Some medical solutions include collagen injections, drug therapy, and using penile clamps or cuffs. Many men choose to have an artificial sphincter surgically implanted.

Talk to your doctor about the many options for dealing with incontinence. Choosing one will give you the freedom to get on with your life the way you used to.

If a man loses his potency,
you dry and crush a male bat that is ready to mate;
you put it into water which has sat out on the roof;
you give it to him to drink; that man will then recover potency.
Ancient Mesopotamian remedy to cure impotence

13

Overcoming impotence: Achieving sexual satisfaction

If you have ever had even one episode of impotence, you know the frustration will drive you to do almost anything to correct the problem. If it's any consolation, men throughout history and all over the world have felt the same.

Around 2000 B.C. in the Mesopotamian area of the world (what is now modern-day Iraq), men with impotence problems relied on Saziga spells — rituals designed to restore potency. They used incantations along with herbal remedies and sometimes even sex organs from animals. Compared to that, modern remedies for impotence are a piece of cake.

When most men hear "prostate" they think "impotence," or to be more politically correct, "erectile dysfunction." Impotence may be the most feared complication of prostate disorders.

Impotence is not usually a symptom of prostate problems. Premature ejaculation or pain during intercourse are the most common sexual symptoms of a prostate disorder. Impotence is more likely to be a side effect of treatment for prostate problems.

Impotence is defined as the inability to experience sexual intercourse, especially because of an inability to have an erection. However, you don't have to have an erection to have an orgasm. An erection occurs just so your penis will be stiff enough to penetrate your mate's vagina. Although impotence can be

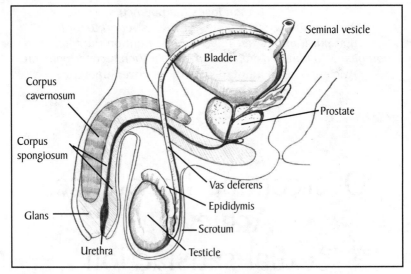

Figure 13.1 - The penis and surrounding organs.

frustrating to you and your mate, it doesn't necessarily mean the death of your sexual enjoyment. There are options that will enable you to enjoy a satisfying sex life.

Erection — your own hydraulic system

Knowing how an erection works helps you understand how it can fail to work, and the best way to explain the process is to compare it to hydraulics. Most men are familiar with the way a hydraulic brake system works. When you apply force to a liquid, like brake fluid, it resists by building up pressure that activates your braking system.

An erection works by the same principle, but instead of brake fluid, your liquid is blood. Two chambers, called the corpora cavernosa, run the length of your penis. When you become sexually stimulated, nerve impulses signal the muscles in these chambers to relax, allowing blood to flow into the space. The extra blood creates pressure, which causes your penis to expand, resulting in an erection.

The problem can occur when your system springs a leak or gets clogged up. Everyone knows what happens when you don't have enough brake fluid in your car. You press the brake pedal and nothing happens (or not enough happens). Impotence occurs when you can't get enough blood flow into your penis. You provide it with stimulation and nothing happens.

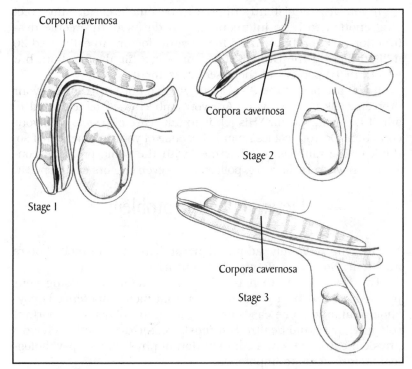

Figure 13.2 - The process of an erection.

Stage 1 - The spongy tissue of the corpora cavernosa contains many blood vessels. These are normally constricted (closed off) so the penis remains soft.

Stage 2 - With sexual stimulation, these blood vessels begin to relax, allowing blood into the penis and causing it to become firmer.

Stage 3 - The corpora cavernosa continue to swell with blood. They press against the penile veins, preventing blood from leaving the penis. With the corpora full of blood, the penis is now firm enough for sexual intercourse.

How to identify impotence

Do you have an erectile dysfunction? In most cases, the answer is pretty obvious, but just because you have difficulty achieving an erection once or twice does not mean you are impotent. Everyone has trouble now and then. Stress, drinking too much alcohol, or fatigue can cause you to have a temporary problem.

If you are consistently unable to become erect or stay erect long enough to have intercourse, you do have an erectile dysfunction, and probably need to see your doctor. An estimated 20 million men in the United States have erectile dysfunction, but less than 10 percent of them seek treatment.

If you are one of the 90 percent who do not try to correct your problem, ask yourself why. Are you embarrassed or ashamed to admit it to your doctor? His job is to take care of people with your condition. Do you feel less manly because of your impotence? If so, think of the millions of other men with the same problem; construction workers, lawyers, policemen — even doctors experience it.

Determining the problem

OK, you've finally admitted it, at least to yourself. You're impotent. Now what do you do about it?

The first step is to figure out what might be causing your problem. It may be a popular notion that most impotence is psychological, and some cases are — your mind plays an important role in your sexual health. But most erectile dysfunctions have a physical cause. Often, a combination of physical and psychological factors leads to impotence.

To determine if your problem may be psychological, take a look at what's been going on in your life and consider the time your problem began. Were you under more stress than usual?

Were you having problems with your relationship, or financial or job difficulties? It may be hard to believe, but stress on the job can affect your performance at home.

Subconscious or even conscious fears may also lead to impotence. For example, some men with cancer worry that tumor cells may in some way be transplanted sexually. Or, they may avoid sex, feeling that some earlier sexual indiscretion caused them to develop prostate problems or cancer in the first place. Other men with cancer avoid sex because they are concerned that increases in hormone levels may cause recurrence of cancer. If any of these fears are interfering with your sex life, put them to bed permanently. They are myths and misconceptions, nothing more.

You can help determine whether your impotence is physical or psychological while you sleep. Your testosterone level peaks about the time the sun rises, which accounts for your penis rising at about the same time. Almost every man experiences this early morning erection. If you are able to have an erection in your sleep, your problem is probably not physical and you should look for ways to eliminate the emotional stress in your life.

An easy way to find out if you have nightly erections is the stamp test. Simply attach a roll of perforated stamps around your flaccid penis before you go to bed. If you have an erection during the night, your growing penis will snap the perforations between the stamps. If you wake up, and your stamps are snapped, that means your blood and nerve supply is enough to achieve an erection. If your stamps are still in one piece, you may want to repeat the test for a couple more nights, but it may mean your impotence has a physical basis.

Physical causes of impotence

Most impotence is caused by physical conditions that reduce blood flow. You cannot achieve an erection without enough blood to fill your penis. Some of the most common physical causes of impotence include:

Alcohol or other addiction. If you smoke, stop. If you drink alcohol, do so only in moderation or quit completely. Both of these habits can restrict blood flow to the penis and make your problems worse.

Diabetes. Diabetic men have a greater risk of becoming impotent. Doctors don't know exactly why, but they think the nerves or blood vessels that control blood flow to your penis may be damaged by diabetes. If you are diabetic, avoiding impotence is a good reason to keep your disorder under control. Follow your diet, exercise regularly, and monitor your blood sugar closely. It could make a difference in your sex life as well as your health.

Prescription drugs. Some drugs cause impotence as a side effect. Medications for high blood pressure and antidepressants are the most common offenders. Check with your doctor or pharmacist if you suspect your prescription may be causing your impotence.

Heart and blood vessel disorders. Since blood flow is so important to achieving an erection, any disorder that interferes with that may cause impotence. Atherosclerosis, a condition in which fatty deposits build up in your blood vessels and restrict blood flow, is a common cause of impotence, especially in older men.

Injury. An injury to your spinal cord can interfere with the nerves you need for an erection. An injury to the penis itself can also cause impotence.

Kidney failure/liver disease. Kidney and liver disorders may affect the hormones you need to become sexually aroused.

Prostate-related impotence

Some men refuse treatment for their prostate problems because they are afraid the treatment will leave them impotent. Some treatments for prostate problems do cause impotence as a side effect, but the risk may be small when compared to the risk of non-treatment.

Finasteride. Finasteride (Proscar) is one of the most prescribed medications for prostate. It works by shrinking your prostate. The problem is, it may also cause your penis to shrink, or at least keep it from expanding when you want it to. According to studies, finasteride is 31 percent effective in reducing BPH symptoms, but it may increase your risk of impotence by 2.5 to 5.3 percent.

Surgery. Any type of pelvic surgery, such as prostate, bladder, colon or rectal surgery, may cause impotence if nerves that affect erection are cut or removed. The percentage of men experiencing impotence following a prostatectomy may be as high as 30 to 90 percent. A radical prostatectomy may affect erection but not sexual drive or ability to have an orgasm. You may need six to 12 months following surgery to recover erectile function, even after a nerve-sparing prostatectomy. (See Chapter 9.) Plenty of practice is important for recovering function, so keep trying.

Radiation treatment. Radiation treatment in the pelvic area for any reason, including prostate cancer, may affect your ability to have an erection. However, it should not affect your sexual drive or your ability to have an orgasm.

Sure-fire ways to recharge and revitalize your sex life

If your prostate treatment does cause you to experience impotence, you still have options that can breathe new spirit into your sex life.

Perk up your potency with pelvic exercises. Kegel exercises were invented for women, but they can also benefit men with erectile dysfunction. For men suffering from impotence because of leaky veins, pelvic floor exercises provide a good alternative to surgery. Leaky veins cause erection problems just as a leaky air valve has problems inflating a tire. The degree of impairment depends on the amount of leakage.

Although some doctors say pelvic muscles don't have any influence on blood flow to the penis, a recent study suggests otherwise. A team of Belgian urologists treated 150 men who suffered from impotence. Some men had operations, and others did special pelvic muscle exercises called Kegels.

One year after treatment, 58 percent of the men who performed the Kegel exercises were completely cured or were so satisfied with their improvement that they did not opt for surgery. Try Kegels for yourself. It certainly can't hurt, and it may help.

Kegel exercises

▶ Identify the pelvic muscles that need exercising. You can do this by stopping and starting the flow of urine several times when using the bathroom.

▶ Tighten the muscles a little at a time. Contract muscles slowly, hold for a count of 10, and relax the muscles slowly.

▶ Repeat these exercises for the anal pelvic muscles. To find these muscles, imagine you're trying to hold back a bowel movement, without tensing your leg, stomach, or buttock muscles.

▶ Practice tightening all pelvic muscles together, moving from back to front.

Start with five repetitions of each exercise three to five times a day. Gradually work up to 20 or 30 repetitions at once.

Get your blood flowing with ginkgo. This herb has been proven to improve blood flow, so if your impotence is caused by reduced blood flow, ginkgo biloba could be the love potion for you. But be patient, you'll need to take at least 240 mg daily for several months to see an improvement.

Go with ginseng — an ancient aphrodisiac. Ginseng is another herb that has a reputation as an aphrodisiac. Although there isn't much scientific evidence to back up its claim to sex fame, some doctors believe it contains compounds that stimulate nerve cells in your penis, helping you to maintain an erection.

Most studies report few, if any, side effects from taking ginseng. Generally, the most common problems are nervousness and excitability. These usually go away after a few days of use. Other reported side effects include insomnia, skin rashes, diarrhea, nausea, and vomiting. If you have high blood pressure or diabetes, you should consult your doctor if you want to take ginseng.

Rev it up with vacuum pumps. This nonsurgical option for treating impotence uses a vacuum to pull blood into the penis. Once fully erect, a rubber ring is placed at the base of the penis to retain the blood until intercourse is completed.

Approved by the American Urological Association, vacuum pumps are generally considered the most cost effective and least invasive option for treating impotence.

Generally, vacuum pumps don't cause any serious side effects. The most common complaints include the interruption of lovemaking, a numb or cool sensation in the penis, and ejaculation discomfort. The good news is that if your impotence is just a temporary side effect of surgery, some studies suggest that using the vacuum pump may speed up your ability to have natural erections again.

Inject to stay erect. Another treatment option approved by the American Urological Association that you may want to consider is the penile self-injection. A shot of medicine designed to dilate blood vessels successfully reverses impotence in 85 to 90 percent of men, except for those with extremely damaged blood vessels.

Injections improve your ability to have an erection by increasing the flow of blood into your penis. Most men are a bit squeamish about sticking a needle into their penis, but the needle is very small, so the discomfort is usually minimal. You will probably receive your first shot in the doctor's office so he can show you the correct way to give yourself the injection. After that, you call the shots.

Once you give yourself the injection, you can expect your erection to last for about an hour. The rate of complications is low. However, side effects do occur and may include pain, bruising, and prolonged erection, also called priaprism. If you have an erection that lasts longer than four hours, see your urologist immediately. This condition needs to be treated quickly. Prolonged erection can cause permanent damage to your penis, so your doctor needs to give you an erection antidote, a drug that constricts blood vessels.

If you are taking an MAO inhibitor, a common type of antidepressant, you shouldn't use injection therapy. Discuss all medications you are taking with your doctor before beginning injections.

Despite the shots' effectiveness, a recent study found that more than half the men taking them stopped within a year. Some men just wanted a more permanent solution to their problem, some were afraid of needles or side effects, and some complained of a lack of sexual spontaneity. Inconvenience could also be a complaint — the drugs usually require mixing and refrigeration.

Insert a pellet for instant success. A transurethral suppository may be a more attractive alternative to injection therapy. It involves the same type of medicine in many injections, alprostadil, but is delivered without a needle. Instead, a pellet of the medicine is inserted into the tip of the penis with an applicator.

This appears to be an effective method. In one study, alprostadil therapy enabled 64.9 percent of the men tested to have sex at home at least once after insertion compared to only 18.6 percent of men in the placebo group.

Side effects include mild penile pain after some applications and prolonged erections.

Try topical cream therapy. A cream that you rub on your penis to induce an erection may be a simple way to counteract impotence. These creams, which include nitroglycerine and minoxidil, are topical vasodilators; they help open up blood vessels in the penis. They may also give your mate a severe headache, so be sure to wear a condom when using the cream. However, if you are one of the people for whom cream works, and you don't mind using a condom, it may be an easy way to rub away impotence.

Confusing yohimbe and yohimbine can be deadly

Many men who have a problem with impotence are reluctant to see their doctor about it. Some of those men may be making a trip to the herb store instead. While many herbs provide safe, natural alternatives to prescription drugs, that may not be the case with some supposed impotence cures.

If you see your doctor for impotence, he may recommend yohimbine, a prescription-only drug that is made from the bark of an African tree. However, your local herb store may offer a similar herbal solution containing yohimbe. Yohimbe has a long-standing reputation as an aphrodisiac, and comes from the same source as yohimbine.

However, according to herbal experts, yohimbe can cause dangerous side effects, including high blood pressure, irregular heartbeat, nausea, and vomiting. An overdose could even lead to paralysis or death.

Yohimbine has been one of the most common drugs pre-scribed for impotence. Although it increases sex drive in rats, its effectiveness in humans has not been totally proven. According to studies, it does have a pronounced placebo effect, which means that people may experience an improvement. Since some cases of impotence are psychological anyway, yohimbine may help by improving your attitude toward sex.

Although prescription yohimbine may not be as dangerous as its cousin yohimbe, it does cause some side effects, including dizziness, nausea, nervousness, and headaches.

Promising new treatment — a pill to make you potent

Wouldn't it be nice if you could just pop a pill and watch your formerly frustrated penis pop up, ready for action? Now you can do just that.

Sildenafil (Viagra) is a drug that was first developed as a treatment for high blood pressure. It didn't work for blood pressure, but the people trying it noticed that it did wonders for their sex lives. Unlike injectable drugs, Viagra doesn't produce an automatic erection — you still need to be "in the mood," but if you're willing, Viagra may help make you able.

In tests, Viagra produced favorable results in 48 to 81 percent of the people who tried it, depending on the severity of their condition. Tests are underway now to see if Viagra can help women with sexual dysfunction.

Recently approved by the FDA, sildenafil is now available with a prescription. Check with your doctor if you think this is the treatment for you.

Surgical solutions to save your sex life

Although some types of surgery, including prostatectomy, can cause impotence, there are also surgical solutions that may reverse erectile dysfunction for many men.

Vascular surgery. This procedure attempts to correct any blood flow problems to and from the penis. The surgery tends to be most successful in healthy young men who have suffered some sort of injury to the penis. However, results appear to be unpredictable for most men. The chances of success are probably not high enough to risk the side effects of major surgery.

Penile implants. Although penile prostheses (implants) are proven to work and have been approved by the American Urological Association, you'll probably want to save this option for last. Once you have a penile implant, it limits your ability to try other options. If surgery caused your impotence, most urologists require that you wait at least a year after surgery before you have a penile implant.

In this technique, a surgeon will insert a semirigid device into your penis that produces either a permanent erection or an erection that can be controlled by using a surgically inserted pump that you can inflate or deflate as you wish.

An implant shouldn't affect your ability to have an orgasm or ejaculate. The sensation in your penis will also be the same as before. You should take four to six weeks to recover from surgery before trying out your new implant.

Penile prostheses can be divided into two basic types — hydraulic and non-hydraulic. The hydraulic prostheses are also called inflatable prostheses, and the non-hydraulic ones are referred to as semirigid rod prostheses or malleable penile prostheses.

▶ **Rod device.** This is the simplest and least expensive version of penile implant. However, because this device cannot be pumped up or deflated on demand, it leads to a constant erection. Some men find this awkward and embarrassing.

Choosing the best treatment

Treatment	Pros
Vacuum devices	Inexpensive; easy-to-use; safe
Injection therapy	Effective
Penile implants	Permanent; reliable
Transurethral suppository	Easy to use; effective
Topical creams	Easy to use; allows spontaneity
Vascular surgery	Restores ability to have normal erection
Yohimbine	Easy to use
Hormone therapy	Easy
Viagra (sildenafil)	Effective; easy to use; allows spontaneity

▶ **Simple self-contained inflatable pump.** This implant allows you more control over erections with a pump that you can use to inflate or deflate your penis as desired. To achieve an erection, you simply squeeze the pump, which then transfers fluid stored in a reservoir into inflated cylinders that have been surgically inserted into your penis. This device practically reproduces a normal erection. However, you may experience problems if the surgery wasn't done exactly right or if the device develops mechanical failure.

▶ **Three-piece inflatable implant.** This device consists of two hollow cylinders, a pump and valve mechanism, and a reservoir. The pump is located in your scrotum, and when you want to have an erection, you simply squeeze the pump several times, which moves fluid into the cylinders. You can easily deflate it by pressing the release valve on the side of the pump. It is more sophisticated than the simple self-contained inflatable pump, and allows you more control as well as increased penis length and girth.

Cons
May cause skin irritation; loss of spontaneity; can injure penis if improperly used
Inconvenient; loss of spontaneity; requires you to give yourself shot; side effects include pain, bruising, build-up of scar tissue, and prolonged erections
Expensive; irreversible
Side effects include penile pain, prolonged erections; not recommended with pregnant partners
Not always effective, must use condom
Expensive, not always effective
Not always effective; side effects include dizziness, nausea, nervousness, and headaches
May cause prostate growth
Circulates in your entire system; does not work for everyone; effectiveness after prostate surgery unknown

Hormonal help may also be harmful

As you get older, you begin to notice certain changes. You have less energy, your hair begins to gray, and your memory starts to slip. Your sexual performance starts to slip, too. It takes longer for you to achieve an erection, it isn't as rock-hard as it used to be, and when you do get an erection, it's more difficult to sustain.

When some men reach this point in their life, they reach for youth in a bottle — hormonal compounds that promise to return their youth and rejuvenate their sex life. Of these compounds, DHEA is probably the most popular.

DHEA is a hormone precursor that is converted into testosterone in your body. As you age, your levels of DHEA decline, which has led some researchers to believe that replenishing your body's supply of it could help turn back the clock.

However, although studies are promising, there is no solid evidence that DHEA can delay or reverse the symptoms of aging, and it may cause your prostate to grow. Only men with low levels of DHEA and normal PSA levels should even consider taking DHEA supplements. If you've had prostate cancer, you should avoid DHEA. If you do decide to take DHEA, you should have your PSA monitored regularly by a doctor.

Master your mind for sexual success

Some psychics claim to be able to raise an object in the air using only their minds. An erection seems to work the same way; you can make your penis rise just by thinking about sex. Unfortunately, the reverse is also true. When you have other things weighing on your mind, you may be unable to perform sexually.

Experts estimate that psychological factors account for 10 to 20 percent of impotence cases. However, even if your impotence has a physical basis, your mind may contribute to your problem. If you have an episode of impotence due to physical causes, drinking too much alcohol for example, you may become embarrassed and anxious, and your next attempt may fail simply because you're so worried about failing.

If your impotence is caused by a serious physical problem, like nerve damage, you need more than positive thinking. However, never underestimate the power of the human mind.

If you have an impotence problem that may be psychological, consider seeing a therapist. Otherwise, learn to relax, lessen the stress in your life, and have confidence that your mind will help make things happen.

In summary

Prostate and impotence do not necessarily go hand in hand. Impotence is usually a side effect of prostate treatment rather than a symptom of prostate disease.

Most impotence has a physical cause, usually restricted blood flow or impaired nerves. Prostate surgery may cause impotence because nerves that control erection may be cut away during the operation.

Even if your prostate treatment leads to impotence, it is usually temporary, and you do have options for dealing with it.

Vacuum pump therapy. This mechanical device works by drawing blood into your penis. One reported benefit is that it may increase your penis size. In fact, some men who don't have an impotence problem use vacuum pumps for that reason.

Injection therapy. While this is a very effective means of achieving erection, you must be willing to give yourself shots in your penis. It is also inconvenient and has potentially serious side effects, including a build-up of scar tissue with repeated use.

Transurethral suppository. Alprostadil is an impotence drug that you deliver into the tip of your penis with a syringe-type applicator.

Oral drugs. Yohimbine has been prescribed for impotence for a long time, but studies find that it's not very effective. A new drug, Viagra, is now on the market. Supposedly, it is very effective with few side effects.

Penile implants. Implants require surgery that removes penile tissue, so it is irreversible. Once you have an implant, you will never be able to have a natural erection again. Several different types of implants are available, ranging from a simple malleable rod to sophisticated hydraulic pump systems.

Topical creams. Creams may be the easiest impotence remedy to use, but they aren't effective for many people and can give your mate a severe headache.

To decide which impotence remedy is right for you, carefully weigh the pros and cons, and discuss all options with your doctor. Rest assured that once you find one you're comfortable with, sex will again be an enjoyable and satisfying part of your life.

This life is a test.
It is only a test.
Had this been your real life
It would have come with further instructions.
Author unknown

14

Diagnostic tests

For a man with prostate problems, all the different tests your doctor is likely to do may seem both perpetual and perplexing. As annoying as they can be, they are important in helping your doctor make an accurate diagnosis so that he can recommend an appropriate treatment. This can mean a faster and easier recovery for you.

This chapter will help you understand the different tests your doctor may do as well as what to expect during the test. You'll also find out whether or not you need to make special preparations for any of the particular tests.

All the tests you may encounter are listed in alphabetical order to help you find them easily. At the end of the chapter, you'll find a section listing recommended tests, optional tests, and unnecessary tests for different prostate disorders. This section can help you determine if your doctor is ordering appropriate tests.

Alkaline phosphatase test (ALP)
Your doctor might order this blood test to determine if prostate cancer has spread outside the prostate into your bones. He will most likely use other tests in addition to the ALP, since conditions besides cancer, as well as drugs and broken bones, can give a high reading.

Bone scan (Radionuclide scintigraphy)
Bone scans are generally thought to be the most sensitive way to spot changes within the bones themselves, usually new

growths of cancer. This is important since prostate cancer will often spread to the bones in the pelvis, hips, back, and thighs.

To perform this scan, you will be given an injection of a harmless, radioactive material. After two to three hours, you will lie on a table while a special camera takes pictures of particular parts of your body. Making the pictures will take 30 to 45 minutes. A radiologist will later read the films, looking for "hot spots" that possibly indicate cancer.

Some experts believe you should have a bone scan as soon as prostate cancer is diagnosed. However, other experts don't believe a bone scan is always necessary after a prostate cancer diagnosis, especially if the PSA is less than 10 ng/mL and the tumor appears to be low grade and low volume.

Chest X-ray

A small percentage of men with prostate cancer will have pieces of the tumor break off and move to the chest or lungs. The later the stage of cancer, the more likely this is to happen. A routine X-ray, following a diagnosis of cancer, can help your doctor watch for this.

Complete blood count

This test measures red blood cells, white blood cells, and platelets. A decrease in normal numbers may indicate cancer has spread to the bones.

Computed tomography (CT or CAT scan)

This scan is a painless, relatively quick way to get pictures of the prostate using X-ray, computer data processing, and mathematics. It cannot show cancer within the prostate, but it can help your doctor check for prostate enlargement.

This test also looks for enlarged lymph nodes and checks to see if the cancer has spread to nearby organs.

Creatinine blood test

Creatinine is filtered out of your blood by your kidneys and then excreted in your urine. If you have high levels of creatinine in your blood, this usually means your kidneys aren't working well. Since quite often, prostate problems affect your kidneys, this is important information for your doctor.

Cystometry

Doctors use this test to aid them in diagnosing prostate enlargement. It involves inserting two small catheters through the urethra and into the bladder. One catheter fills the bladder with water or carbon dioxide gas while the other catheter records pressure changes in the bladder while it is being filled and emptied. There is a chance you could develop a urinary tract infection after this procedure, so be sure and keep your doctor informed of problems or fever.

Cystoscopy

See Urethrocystoscopy

Digital rectal exam (DRE)

To check your prostate, the doctor will ask you to undress and bend over. He will then insert a gloved, lubricated finger about 4 inches into your rectum and press down. Although this exam is uncomfortable, it should not cause you any actual pain. (Doctors who have had the exam themselves vouch for this.)

During the rectal exam, your doctor will try to determine if your prostate has any hard lumps, which may suggest cancer, or if any areas feel tender and soft, which may indicate infection. If your doctor suspects an infection, he will probably want to do a urine test. For the most accurate diagnosis, most doctors use the segmented urine culture.

Intravenous pyelogram (IVP)

This is an X-ray of your urinary system. It helps the doctor determine if you have any problems with your urinary tract or kidneys. In order to make your kidneys, bladder, and ureters visible on the X-ray screen, the doctor injects your veins with a dye that gathers in those areas. You should not have this test if you are allergic to iodine.

Magnetic resonance imaging (MRI)

An MRI is a safe but expensive procedure used only if you have already been diagnosed with prostate cancer. It gives your doctor pictures that let him see how far the cancer has spread. He then uses this information to plan treatment or surgery.

During this half-hour test, you lie on a table that rolls into a small scanning chamber. Here, a magnetic field causes the atoms in your body to give off electromagnetic energy. This energy is read as radio waves that are then turned into images.

Some people experience claustrophobia when they are inside the chamber. For this reason, many facilities have music or even television to help take your mind off your surroundings. If necessary, you can be sedated.

Medical history

Your doctor will ask you questions about your symptoms, previous medical problems, and about any habits he feels may be contributing to your problem. He'll want to know about surgeries and medications. Family history can be especially important, so research any medical problems your father, grandfather, brothers, or uncles have.

Learning about your job and your hobbies may give him some useful information as well. He may ask specific questions about your sexual and urinary habits. Try not to feel self-conscious about these. Just give him honest, complete answers. Remember to take all medical records and any written logs you have of your symptoms, and don't be afraid to ask questions.

Pelvic lymph node dissection

If none of the other tests offer a definite conclusion as to whether cancer has spread to the lymph nodes, the urologist may remove a lymph node from your body and examine it to make a determination. It can be done by laparoscopic surgery, a procedure where tiny holes are made beneath the navel to remove the lymph nodes, rather than through a large incision. Most men have a much faster recovery time with laparoscopic surgery— some are even doing it as outpatients.

It is also acceptable to remove the lymph nodes through a small incision in your lower abdomen. This procedure may be performed at the same time as a planned prostate operation.

Physical exam

A physical exam is necessary so your doctor can get an idea of your general health. He will take your height, weight, temperature, heart rate, and blood pressure. You might also need to

give a blood sample for other tests. Finally, your doctor will probably poke and prod your stomach and pelvic areas to check for
swollen or tender spots.

Pressure-flow study

This test measures the pressure in your bladder as you urinate. That number is then compared to the speed of your urine
stream. Some doctors feel this test is the best way to find out
how much your urination ability is blocked.

To perform the pressure-flow study, a small tube called a
catheter is inserted into your penis, through the urethra, and
into the bladder. The test may cause discomfort for a short time.
In a few men, it may cause a urinary tract infection.

Prostascint

This test detects prostate cancer cells that have spread. The
procedure has the potential to prevent a lot of unnecessary radical prostatectomies. The prostascint can predict with 68 percent
accuracy if a cancer has spread outside your prostate or not.
That means you may be able to avoid a radical prostatectomy
and two of the common complications that often accompany that
procedure — incontinence and impotence.

Because this test can pinpoint whether cancer has spread to
your lymph nodes or bones, it can help determine which type of
management program would benefit you most. For example, if
your prostate cancer has spread to the lymph nodes in your
pelvis, the ideal treatment is radiation therapy. If the cancer has
spread to lymph nodes in the abdominal area, hormonal therapy would probably be best.

Prostate biopsy

To determine if cancer is present in your prostate, your doctor will insert a long hollow needle into your prostate by way of
your rectum or your perineum (the area between the anus and
the penis). The needle removes a small core of prostate tissue.
Mildly uncomfortable, this procedure takes about 20 minutes.

Prostate specific antigen (PSA) test

A normal prostate regularly produces the protein PSA. Slightly higher PSA levels in your blood may suggest benign prostatic

hyperplasia (BPH). That means the prostate is enlarging and producing more of this protein. The higher the PSA levels, the more likely it is that cancer is present in the prostate.

This simple blood test measures PSA levels and tells your doctor if there is reason to suspect you have prostate cancer or BPH. But a number of things can make the test results inaccurate. One problem is that prostates vary in size and, therefore, will produce different amounts of PSA. Doctors are working to come up with standards for healthy PSA levels for different age groups so they can better analyze test results. Even with its inaccuracies, the PSA test is still the most useful screening test in the field.

To avoid skewing results, you should not have this test for 48 to 72 hours after a rectal exam. For the same reason, you should also avoid sex for at least two days before this test.

According to the American Cancer Society and the American Urological Association, if you are over 40 and in a high-risk group, or over 50, you should have a PSA test annually.

Prostatic acid phosphatase (PAP)

This test has long been used to measure how much acid phosphatase, an enzyme secreted by the prostate, has leaked into your bloodstream. Too much can mean something is wrong, possibly that cancer has spread to your lymph nodes or other parts of your body. However, other conditions or procedures, such as prostatic infarction or prostate massage, can also cause your serum acid phosphatase (ACP) level to rise. In many cases this test is not sensitive enough to give your doctor really helpful information. For these reasons, this test is usually requested only after there is evidence of prostate cancer, for example after a tissue biopsy.

PSA density

One of the reasons the PSA test can give incorrect results is because prostates come in all sizes. A broad rule is that larger prostates produce more PSA than smaller ones. Therefore, a high PSA reading could simply mean you have a large, but normal, prostate.

To fix this problem with the PSA test, doctors measure the size or volume of your prostate with a transrectal ultrasound and divide the PSA by this number. The result is your PSA density, or the amount of PSA produced per gram of prostate.

PSA, free vs. bound

PSA exists in two forms: free and bound. One way doctors can more clearly determine whether or not cancer is actually present is by comparing the amount of free PSA to total PSA.

These two types of PSA are identified by whether or not they are attached to a protein. Free or unbound PSA is not attached to a protein; bound PSA is attached to a protein. A low percent of free PSA and a high percent of bound PSA suggest cancer.

If this test is approved by the FDA (and it looks as though it probably will be in the near future), it could potentially save needless anxiety and discomfort for almost 1 million men per year. In addition, it could save the cost of performing a biopsy if the regular PSA test is high.

This test could be especially beneficial for African-American men, whose cancers are less likely to be detected using standard PSA ranges.

PSA velocity

If your doctor wants to monitor your PSA, you might have to go in for repeat tests every so often. He will then measure how much and how quickly your PSA levels rise. This is a good way to tell if there is cancer and if it is growing.

Residual urine measurement

This test often follows uroflowmetry and is designed to show if the bladder empties normally or not. A catheter is inserted into the bladder to empty and measure any remaining urine. Today, most doctors prefer to use ultrasound to estimate residual urine.

Reverse transcriptase polymerase chain reaction (RT)-PCR

In order for your doctor to prescribe the correct treatment, he must know if the cancer is limited to the prostate or if it has spread to other places in your body. The (RT)-PCR is a very sensitive test that looks for cancer cells in your blood. It can help distinguish between cases of prostate cancer that will spread and require treatment from those that will remain dormant.

However, (RT)-PCR is still rather new and experimental and is not yet used routinely.

Segmented urine culture

If your doctor suspects a prostate problem, he may request a segmented urine culture (also called the Meares and Stamey test). If you know in advance you're going to have this test or even think you may, it's best not to ejaculate two to three days before your appointment as it may skew the test results. Ejaculation normally leaves your prostate slightly inflamed. Also, be sure to drink plenty of water on the day of your appointment.

For the test, you will be given four sterile cups. You will be asked to release enough urine to cover the bottom of the first cup. For your midstream sample, you will be asked to urinate a little more (but not all yet) into the second cup.

Before you urinate into the third cup, your doctor will do a prostatic massage. With a gloved finger inserted into your rectum, he will stroke your prostate six to seven times on each side. This often stimulates a few drops of the prostate secretion to come out of the tip of the penis. If nothing appears, you force out the secretions by urinating into the fourth cup. (Now you see why it's important to drink a lot of water before your appointment. You're going to need it!)

All samples will be sent to the lab for a special culture test to determine if bacteria are present and if so what kind. If bacteria are found in either of the first two cups you urinated in, you have a urethral or bladder infection. Bacteria in the last two cups indicates a prostate infection.

Transrectal ultrasonography (TRUS)

Ultrasound is an important way of seeing various internal organs. The procedure has been around for years, but only recently has a more sophisticated technique been developed that allows doctors to get a good, close-up view of the prostate.

Transrectal ultrasound is different from a normal ultrasound in that a special probe is inserted into the rectum, and very high frequency sound waves are aimed at your prostate. Because the waves pass through different organs at different rates (depending on organ size), the machine creates a general outline of the size and shape of your prostate. The doctor is then able to view your entire prostate, looking for any masses or abnormalities.

Ultrasound is used to look for prostate cancer, usually after a DRE or a high PSA test, and to pinpoint the stage of cancer in those already diagnosed. It can help measure the size and weight of your prostate, which is necessary to come up with a PSA density. Urologists also use ultrasound to guide them during a needle biopsy to make sure they sample the right tissue.

Ultrasound
See Transrectal ultrasonography (TRUS).

Urethrocystoscopy
Using a tool called a cytoscope, your doctor looks directly into your bladder to check for any problems there or in your urethra. He can also see if prostate enlargement is causing your troubles or if cancer has moved into your bladder or is pressing on your urethra.

You will need to completely empty your bladder before the test begins. The doctor must insert the cystoscope through the penis tip and up your urethra to see into the bladder. A special solution numbs the inside of the penis so the procedure is not too uncomfortable. A few men experience urinary infections or blood in the urine after this test. Also, some men are not able to urinate for a short time after the test.

Urinalysis
This test is used to determine whether or not an infection is present. You simply urinate into a plastic cup and the lab then tests your urine for infection or other problems by using a chemically treated plastic stick called a dip stick. The strip will turn different colors depending on what's in your urine. The presence of white blood cells usually indicates an infection. Red blood cells suggest cancer.

Urine cytology test
Used to test for cancer, this test works best if you provide your first urine of the day. Morning urine contains a higher concentration of cells from the bladder wall since it has been in the bladder overnight.

Uroflowmetry (flow rate)
Also called the uroflow test, this test can help clarify whether your problems are indeed caused by an enlarged prostate or by something else.

For this test, you need to have a full bladder. You urinate into a special toilet, which measures how much urine you pass and records the speed of your urine stream. This test is often followed by the residual urine test.

Urogram
See Intravenous pyelogram (IVP).

Diagnosing the different disorders

Listed below are the prostate disorders discussed in this book and the tests doctors normally use to diagnose those conditions. The tests are listed in the order in which the doctor would normally do them. There is likely to be some variation from doctor to doctor, but if your doctor appears to order tests haphazardly or suggests tests that are commonly considered unnecessary or outdated, you may want to consider finding another doctor.

Prostatitis

- Medical history

- Physical exam

- Digital rectal exam (DRE)

- Urine culture (Segmented urine culture)

- Prostatic ultrasound (Transrectal ultrasonography or TRUS)

- Kidney X-ray or ultrasound (Intravenous pyelogram or IVP). This test is usually unnecessary.

- Urethrocystoscopy (Cystoscopy)

- Biopsy. Not normally done to diagnose prostatitis.

Acute bacterial prostatitis

- Medical history

- Physical exam

- Blood test

- Urine culture

- Digital rectal exam (DRE)

- Prostate massage. Should not generally be done as it can spread the infection.

Benign prostatic hyperplasia

Recommended tests:

- Medical history

- Symptom assessment test. To objectively determine how much your symptoms bother you, the Agency for Health Care Policy and Research (AHCPR) suggests you take the International Prostate Screening Score (IPSS), an easy self-test of seven questions. See page 78 for a look at this test.

- Physical exam

- Digital rectal exam (DRE)

- Urinalysis

- Creatinine measurement

Optional tests:

- Prostate specific antigen (PSA) test. This test is optional because it is not a very reliable way to determine if your problems are caused by benign prostatic hyperplasia or prostate cancer. Many times this test comes up "false-positive" (meaning it finds prostate cancer that's really not there) and leads to unnecessary prostate biopsies.

- Uroflowmetry

- Pressure-flow study

- Residual urine measurement

- Urethrocystoscopy. Optional during later evaluation if invasive treatment is being planned.

Unnecessary tests:

- Ultrasonography or urogram

- Cystometry

- Urethrocystoscopy. Not recommended as a procedure to determine the need for treatment.

Optional tests before surgery for BPH

- Uroflow (Uroflowmetry)

- Residual urine test

- Pressure flow studies

- Urethrocystoscopy

Screening tests for cancer

These tests help your doctor determine if you have cancer or not:

- Digital rectal exam (DRE)

- Prostate specific antigen (PSA) test

- Free vs. bound PSA

- PSA velocity

- Transrectal ultrasonography (TRUS)

- Biopsy

Cancer

A number of tests can help your doctor determine where the cancer is:

- Prostate specific antigen (PSA) test

- Bone scan

- Computed tomography (CT or CAT scan)

- Magnetic resonance imaging (MRI)

- Prostascint

- Prostatic acid phosphatase (PAP)

- Alkaline phosphatase test (ALP)

- Pelvic lymph node dissection

- Chest X-ray

- Urethrocystoscopy (Cystoscopy)

- Reverse transcriptase polymerase chain reaction (RT)-PCR

As new diagnostic tests are continually being developed, you may run into some not discussed here. If that's the case, be sure to ask your doctor to explain the test, what it diagnoses, and what you can expect to happen during the test. Also, be sure to ask if you need to follow any special instructions before taking the test.

Although few men look forward to prostate tests, most find them valuable in guiding them and their doctor in choosing the most appropriate treatment. In the end, these tests can point the way to a generally healthier prostate.

There are no foolish questions, and no man becomes a fool until he has stopped asking questions.
Charles P. Steinmetz, electrical engineer and inventor

I5

Organizations and support groups

Prostate disorders may have been an ignored problem in the past, but no more! No matter what's plaguing your prostate, you should be able to find a support group or an organization offering more information listed below. Prostate conditions are listed alphabetically to make searching easier.

Don't hesitate to tap into this valuable network of resources that can provide just the support and information you and your family need to make coping with a prostate problem easier.

Benign prostatic hyperplasia (BPH)

American Foundation for Urologic Disease, Inc.
1128 North Charles Street
Baltimore, MD 21201
(800) 242-2383
admin@afud.org (E-mail)
http://www.access.digex.net/~afud/research.html

This nonprofit organization is dedicated to preventing and curing urologic diseases.

National Kidney and Urologic Diseases Information Clearinghouse
3 Information Way
Bethesda, MD 20892

(301) 654-4415
(301) 468-6345
nkudic@aerie.com (E-mail)
http://www.niddk.nih.gov/health/kidney/nkudic.htm

A division of the National Institutes of Health, this organization provides information on benign prostatic hyperplasia (BPH) and prostatitis. It also makes referrals to urologic organizations.

Brachytherapy

Amersham Healthcare
(800) 228-0126

Manufacturers of Iodine 125, used in brachytherapy. They provide information on brachytherapy, also called seeding, as well as the names of doctors in your area who perform this procedure.

Theragenics Corporation
5325 Oak Brook Parkway
Norcross, GA 30093
(800) 458-4372
(404) 381-4372

Manufactures the seeds used in brachytherapy, also called interstitial radiation therapy treatment of prostate cancer. They also provide general information on radiation therapy as well as the names of doctors in your area who perform this procedure.

Cryosurgery

Society of Urologic Cryosurgeons
(714) 550-9155

Hospice care

Foundation for Hospice and Home Care
513 C Street N.E.
Stanton Park

Washington, DC 20002
(202) 547-6586

Hospice Education Institute
190 Westbrook Road
Essex, CT 06426
(800) 331-1620

National Hospice Organization
1901 North Moore Street, Suite 901
Arlington, VA 22209
(800) 658-8898

National Institute for Jewish Hospice
8723 Alden Drive, Suite 652
Los Angeles, CA 90048
(800) 446-4448

Hospital accreditation

Joint Commission on Accreditation of Healthcare Organizations
One Renaissance Boulevard
Oak Brook Terrace, IL 60181
(708) 916-5600

Living wills

Choice in Dying
200 Varick Street
New York, NY 10014
(800) 989-WILL

Incontinence

Continence Restored, Inc.
407 Strawberry Hill Avenue
Stamford, CT 06902
(914) 285-1470 (daytime)
(203) 348-0601 (evening)

Their mission is to disseminate information about bladder control problems to all interested parties, to establish a network of continence support groups throughout the United States, to provide a resource for the public and professionals, and to work with manufacturers who produce incontinence products.

Home Delivery Incontinent
(800) 538-1036

Offers a catalog of products for incontinence that are delivered straight to your home.

Kimberly-Clark Home Health Care
P.O. Box 2002
Neenah, WI 54956-9002
(800) 242-6463 (Inside Wisconsin)
(800) 558-6423 (Outside Wisconsin)

They manufacture incontinence products and can provide general information on incontinence as well as answer specific questions.

National Association for Continence
(Formerly called Help for Incontinent People, Inc.)
P.O. Box 8310
Spartanburg, SC 29305
(800) BLADDER or (800) 252-3337

Their mission is to improve the quality of life for people with incontinence. They are a leading source of education, advocacy, and support to the public and to the health profession about the causes, prevention, diagnosis, treatment, and management alternatives for incontinence. They offer a newsletter, biennial directory of products and services for incontinence, and assorted educational leaflets on topics related to incontinence. This organization also offers a Continence Referral Service, market research, and information clearinghouse services.

The International Foundation of Bowel Dysfunction
P.O. Box 17864
Milwaukee, WI 53217
(414) 964-1799

The Procter & Gamble Co.
Procter & Gamble Plaza
Cincinnati, OH 45202
(800) 432-4000 (general information)
(800) 4-ATTEND (to receive a product sample)

Provides information and free samples of the company's incontinence products.

The Simon Foundation for Continence
P.O. Box 815
Wilmette, IL 60091
(800) 23-SIMON or (800) 237-4666

Their mission is to remove the stigma from incontinence and provide help to sufferers, their families, and the professional caregiver. They offer a newsletter and other educational materials.

Impotence

American Association of Sex Educators, Counselors, and Therapists (AASECT)
435 North Michigan Avenue, Suite 1717
Chicago, IL 60611
(312) 644-0828

This is a professional organization for sex educators, counselors, and therapists. They maintain a national register of individuals meeting professional standards for membership. If desired, they will refer you to a sex therapist within your area.

Impotence Foundation
(800) 221-5517

Provides general information on treating impotence.

Impotence Information Center
American Medical Systems
11001 Bren Road East

Minnetonka, MN 55343
(800) 543-9632

Impotence Information Center
P.O. Box 9
Minneapolis, MN 55440
(800) 843-4315

Part of the large pharmaceutical company, Pfizer. Manufactures medical devices, including penile implants. Offers free information on causes and treatments of impotence. Also provides names of urologists and support groups in your area.

Impotence Institute of America, Inc.
2020 Pennsylvania Avenue, N.W., Suite 292
Washington, DC 20006
(800) 669-1603

Provides information on impotence as well as a list of doctors who treat it. Also sponsors a support group called Impotence Anonymous and a sister support group for partners of men with impotence.

Impotence World Association
1400 Little Patuxent Parkway, Suite 485
Columbia, MD 21044-3502
(800) 669-1603
(410) 715-9605

Their mission is to inform and educate the public about impotence and its causes and treatments and to maintain a referral list of urologists who will treat and diagnose impotence. The following information is available by contacting them: *Not All In Your Head* (book), *Impotence Worldwide* (newsletter), Impotence: Help and Hope (videotape).

Information Center
American Medical Systems
Minneapolis, MN 55440
(800) 543-9632

American Medical Systems is one of the leading manufacturers of medical devices designed to help men cope with and overcome impotence. They also manufacture artificial sphincters and the equipment needed to perform a balloon dilation. They offer free information to the general public on impotence and incontinence.

Not for Men Only
Mercy Hospital and Medical Center
Stevenson Expressway at King Drive
Chicago, IL 60616
(312) 567-5567

An impotence support group for men and their partners.

Palisades Pharmaceutical, Inc.
64 North Summit Street
Tenafly, NJ 07670
(800) 237-9083

They manufacture a yohimbine drug sold under the trade name Yocon. Also offer information on the drug and where you can receive yohimbine treatment.

Potency Restored
Dr. Guilio Scarzella
Montgomery Center, Suite 218
8630 Fenton Street
Silver Spring, MD 20910
(301) 588-5777

An impotence support group for couples.

Recovery of Male Potency (ROMP)
ROMP Center
Grace Hospital
18700 Meyers Road
Detroit, MI 48235
(800) TEL ROMP
(313) 927-3219

Support group for men with erectile dysfunction that meets at medical centers around the country. Approximately 25 ROMP support groups operate throughout the United States.

Sexual Function Health Council
American Foundation for Urologic Disease, Inc.
300 West Pratt Street, Suite 401
Baltimore, MD 21201
(800) 242-2383

SIECUS (Sexuality Information and Education Council of the United States)
130 West 42nd Street, Suite 350
New York, NY 10036
(212) 819-9770

Provides information on illness and sexuality.

Star Center
27211 Lahser Road, Suite 208
Southfield, MI 48034
(800) 835-7667
(313) 357-1314

Provides general information on impotence and makes referrals to doctors in your area.

The Geddings Osbon, Sr. Foundation
P.O. Box 1593
Augusta, GA 30903-1593
(800) 433-4215
Impotence@gdo.org (E-mail)
http://www.impotence.org/

Osborn Medical Systems
P.O. Box 1478
Augusta, GA 30903
(800) 438-8592

They manufacture external vacuum devices, offer free information on all aspects of impotence, and can make referrals to specialists within your area. They also offer educational booklets and slide/video programs for consumers and medical professionals.

Infertility

Resolve, Inc.
1310 Broadway
Somerville, MA 02144
(617) 623-1156

Insurance

The National Coalition for Cancer Survivorship
1010 Wayne Avenue
Silver Spring, MD 20910
(301) 585-2626
(301) 650-8868

Offers information and help on practical insurance matters for people with cancer.

Health Care Financing Administration, Office of Public Affairs
U.S. Department of Health and Human Services
Hubert H. Humphrey Building, Room 435-H
200 Independence Avenue S.W.
Washington, DC 20001
(202) 690-6113
Medicare hotline (800) 638-6833

Medical records

American Health Information Management Association
Office of Legislative Affairs
919 North Michigan Avenue, Suite 1400
Chicago, IL 60611
(312) 787-2672

Offers assistance if you are having problems with your medical records.

Pain

American Pain Society
5700 Old Orchard Road
Skokie, IL 60077
(708) 966-5595

International Pain Foundation
909 Northeast 43rd Street, Suite 306
Seattle, WA 98105-6020
(206) 547-2157

American Chronic Pain Association
P.O. Box 850
Rocklin, CA 95677
(916) 632-0922
ACPA@pacbell.net (E-mail)

This organization provides a support system for people suffering with chronic pain.

National Chronic Pain Outreach Association
7979 Old Georgetown Road, Suite 100
Bethesda, MD 20814
(301) 652-4948

Prostate cancer

American Cancer Society
1599 Clifton Road, N.E.
Atlanta, GA 30329-4251
(800) ACS-2345
(404) 320-3333
http://www.cancer.org

Provides information and financial assistance in some cases to help people who are coping with various cancers, including prostate cancer. Offers the free brochure "Facts on Prostate Cancer." The American Cancer Society also sponsors a nationwide network of support groups called Man to Man. Call to find the location of a group near you. Some groups also offer a support session for women partners of men with prostate cancer called Side by Side.

American Institute for Cancer Research
1759 R Street, N.W.
Washington, DC 20009
(800) 843-8114 (Nutrition Hotline and Cancer Resource Requests)
aicrweb@aicr.org (E-mail)
http://www.aicr.org

This organization offers information on diet, nutrition, and cancer. It also has information available on cancer prevention.

American Foundation for Urologic Disease, Inc.
Prostate Cancer Support Network
300 West Pratt Street, Suite 401
Baltimore, MD 21201-2463
(800) 242-2383
(800) 828-7866

They offer a free booklet, "Prostate Cancer: What Every Man Over 40 Should Know," and other materials on cancer and non-cancerous prostate conditions.

American Society of Clinical Oncology
225 Reinekers Lane
Suite 650
Alexandria, VA 22314
(703) 299-0150
http://www.asco.org

Professional members of this society conduct clinical cancer research. This organization also offers scientific and educational information.

Canadian Cancer Society
10 Alcorn Avenue, Suite 200
Toronto, Ontario
Canada M4V 3B1
(416) 961-7223

Offers information and support to people with cancer.

Cancer Care, Inc.
1180 Avenue of the Americas
New York, NY 10036
(800) 813-HOPE
(212) 221-3300
(212) 302-2400 (social services)
Info@cancercareinc.org (E-mail)
http://www.cancercareinc.org

Offers professional counseling, education, support group information, and help with practical problems.

Cancer Hot Line
R.A. Bloch Cancer Foundation, Inc.
4410 Main Street
Kansas City, MO 64111
(816) WE-BUILD or (816) 932-8453

Provides information and referrals for people with cancer.

Cancer Support Network
5895 Devereau Lane
Pittsburgh, PA 15232
(412) 661-8949

Offers educational programs and support groups for people with cancer and their families.

CaP Cure (Association for the Cure of Cancer of the Prostate)
1250 Fourth Street, Suite 360
Santa Monica, CA 90401
(310) 458-2873
(800) 757-CURE

Founded by financier Michael Milken to find a cure for prostate cancer. Upon request, CaP Cure will send a list of funded research projects.

Make Today Count
(800) 432-2273

A support group for men with prostate cancer. Call to find the location of a group near you.

The Mathews Foundation for Prostate Cancer Research
1010 Hurley Way, Suite 195
Sacramento, CA 95825
(800) 234-6284

Compiles information from the media and tailors it to your particular needs. Offers videotapes, books, and telephone counseling.

National Cancer Institute Cancer Information Service
9000 Rockville Pike
Bethesda, MD 20892
(800) 4-CANCER or (800) 422-6237
http://www.nci.nih.gov/hpage/cis.htm

This organization provides free cancer information to anyone who requests it. In addition to general booklets on prostate cancer, they also provide a computer printout of the status of the latest clinical trials and other treatments currently under investigation by the National Cancer Institute. If you have cancer, they encourage you to show the clinical trial data to your doctor. You can also speak with a cancer information specialist.

National Coalition for Cancer Survivorship
1010 Wayne Avenue
Silver Spring, MD 20910-5600
(301) 650-8868

Provides the names of national support groups and offers information about health insurance and work rights.

National Hospice Organization
1910 North Fort Meyer Drive, Suite 307
Arlington, VA 22209
(800) 658-8898

They can help you locate a hospice in your area.

Patient Advocates for Advanced Cancer Treatments (PAACT), Inc.
1143 Parmelee, N.W.
Grand Rapids, MI 49504
(616) 453-1477

A nonprofit, membership organization incorporated in 1987, PAACT provides information on treatments for advanced prostate cancer. As a member, you receive the *Prostate Cancer Report*, a monthly newsletter, and access to a telephone service that offers prerecorded reports on prostate cancer. They work to speed up drug approval procedures by the Food and Drug Administration (FDA). Especially active in promoting hormone therapy, cryosurgery, and other alternative treatments for prostate cancer.

Prostate Cancer Communication Resource, Inc.
P.O. Box 6023
Carefree, AZ 85377
(602) 488-1915

This nonprofit organization offers "Magic of the Mind," by Larry Becker, a magician, mentalist, and prostate cancer survivor.

Prostate Cancer Resource Network
P.O. Box 966
New Port Richey, FL 34656
(813) 847-1619
(800) 915-1001

A charitable foundation, Prostate Cancer Resource Network provides information, hope, and encouragement to men with prostate cancer and their families. Also provides Survivor's Guide booklets.

US-TOO, International, Inc.
930 N. York Road, Suite 50
Hinsdale, IL 60521
(800) 80-US TOO (800) 808-7866
(708) 323-1002
http://www.ustoo.com

A network of support groups for men with prostate cancer and BPH and their families. US-TOO publishes the *Prostate Cancer Communicator* newsletter and provides information on prostate cancer treatments. They can also give you information on the chapter nearest you.

The Wellness Community
2716 Ocean Park Blvd., Suite 1040
Santa Monica, CA 90405-5211
(310) 314-2555

This support program, which sponsors communities throughout the United States, offers free psychological and emotional support to people with cancer as well as their families. They can direct you to a community near you.

Prostate problems (general)

American Prostate Society
1340 Charwood Road, Suite F
Hanover, MD 21076
(410) 859-3735
(800) 678-1238

They provide brochures on prostate problems, as well as a quarterly newsletter, and sponsor educational programs.

American Foundation for Urologic Disease, Inc.
300 West Pratt Street, Suite 401
Baltimore, MD 21201
(800) 242-2383
(410) 727-2908

This foundation educates the general public on urological problems and encourages research in the field of urology. It also publishes *Family Urology* and provides information on BPH, prostate cancer, prostate infections, and other problems.

American Urological Association
1120 North Charles Street

Baltimore, MD 21201
(410) 727-1100
(410) 223-4310

A professional society founded in 1902 to represent doctors specializing in urologic disorders in the United States, Canada, Mexico, Central America, and the Pacific and Caribbean regions. They publish the *Journal of Urology.*

National Kidney and Urologic Diseases Information Clearinghouse
Box NKUDIC
9000 Rockville Pike
Bethesda, MD 20892
(301) 654-4415
(301) 468-6345

A division of the National Institutes of Health, this organization provides information on BPH and prostatitis.

Prostate Health Council
American Foundation for Urologic Disease, Inc.
300 W. Pratt Street, Suite 401
Baltimore, MD 21201
(800) 242-2383

Prostatitis

The Prostatitis Foundation Information Distribution Center
Parkway Business Center
2029 Ireland Grove Road
Bloomington, IL 61704
(309) 664-6222
http://www.fullfeed.com/prosfnd or http://www.prostate.org

Provides support to men with prostatitis and pushes for prostatitis research funding. For more information, request The Prostatitis Foundation information packet.

American Board of Urology
31700 Telegraph Road, Suite 150

Bingham Farms, MI 48025
(248) 646-9720

Identifies for the public's knowledge those physicians who have satisfied the Board's criteria for certification and recertification in the specialty of urology.

American Prostate Society
1340-F Charwood Road
Hanover, MD 21076
(410) 859-3735

Their goal is to increase knowledge of prostate diseases and encourage the establishment of centers for diagnosis and treatment. The following brochures are available from them: "What You Don't Know About Your Prostate Can Kill You" and "Medication Versus Surgery." They also publish a quarterly newsletter.

Radical prostatectomy

Prostate Health Council
American Foundation for Urologic Disease, Inc.
300 West Pratt Street
Baltimore, MD 21201
(800) 242-2383

Transportation assistance

Corporate Angel Network
(914) 328-1313

This organization provides volunteer corporate aircraft services to people who need transportation between home and a cancer center. If you would like to use this service, call to register.

*A miracle drug is any drug
that will do what the label says it will do.*
Eric Hodgins, American author, editor, and publisher

16

Commonly prescribed drugs for prostate problems

Using prescription drugs safely

This chapter will answer many of your questions about medications for prostate problems, but it may not give you all the information you want. It's important to communicate with your doctor and get as much information as you can about any drug before you start taking it. Here's a list of questions you should ask your doctor when he prescribes a drug.

What is this drug supposed to do for me?

How long will it take to work?

How often will I need to take it? If I am supposed to take my medicine several times a day, does that mean during my waking hours or at regular intervals, even at night?

What are the drug's side effects? Be sure to note any side effects you experience, no matter how minor they seem. When you experience side effects, your doctor may decide to change the dose, try another drug, stop the medication, or decide the benefits of the drug outweigh the bad effects you are feeling. However, you should never make that decision for yourself. Just as you should never take a drug without your doctor's consent, you should never stop taking prescribed medication without consulting him.

Are there any special cautions because of my age? The older you become, the less efficient your liver and kidneys are at eliminating drugs from your bloodstream. That means drugs stay in your body longer and build up to higher levels than they would in the body of a younger person.

Could this drug aggravate other medical conditions I already have?

Are there other drugs that may interact with my prescription? Let your doctor know about all other drugs you take, even over-the-counter cough and cold remedies. Many drugs interact with each other, increasing or decreasing the desired effects. Interactions may be visible changes, or they may be measurable only by laboratory tests.

Are there any foods I shouldn't eat? Some vitamin supplements, foods, and beverages can interact with drugs and change their effects.

How should I store the drug? Most drugs need to be stored in a cool, dry place. Some must be kept cold, and some must be kept away from light. Get specific instructions from your pharmacist if your doctor doesn't know.

Should I take my prescription with or without food or water? Some pills, such as antibiotics, are best taken on an empty stomach. Most pills can be taken with a glass of water to help wash them all the way down your throat and to aid in absorption. Some pills are better taken with food to help avoid stomach irritation, such as the nonsteroidal anti-inflammatory drugs (NSAIDs) like ibuprofen and aspirin. Never take your medicine with hot drinks like tea or coffee because heat can destroy a drug's effectiveness.

What about missed doses? You should normally take all of your prescription, down to the last pill or dose. With some drugs, such as antibiotics, you may start to feel better in a day or two, but that doesn't mean the illness is completely gone. Find out what you should do if you miss a dose of your medication. Sometimes you should make up a missed dose, but sometimes it is safer to skip it and resume your schedule at the next dose time.

Prescription drug cautions

Prescription drugs can provide comfort and cures, but they can also be dangerous if not handled properly. Here are some tips to keep your prescriptions both safe and effective.

Prevent pharmacy errors. As soon as you get your prescription filled, read the label. Then repeat back to the pharmacist the name of the drug and the condition it was prescribed to treat, just to clarify that no mistake has been made. Get the pharmacist to acknowledge that your statement is correct. Then read the instructions for taking the drug. If anything differs from your doctor's instructions to you, or if there is anything you don't understand, ask the pharmacist or call your doctor immediately. Try to find a pharmacist you like and stick with him. He will become an ally who knows some of your medical history. A good relationship with your pharmacist may mean extra attention to your needs and less chance of mix-ups.

Avoid confusion. Because some drugs can be very dangerous if taken by the wrong person, be aware of who in your household may have access to your prescription. Make sure there is no confusion between two different prescriptions that look alike. There are many drugs with very similar names but dramatically different effects.

Never take more than the recommended dosage of any drug. You may just need to give the drug time to accumulate in your body before you notice any good effects. Many drugs can cause dangerous or even fatal side effects if you take too much.

If you accidentally overdose, contact your doctor immediately. If you need hospital or ambulance emergency care, give the medical personnel the medicine bottle so they'll know exactly how to treat you. If the bottle is not available, tell them the exact name and dosage of the drug and the name of the doctor who prescribed it.

Prepare for emergencies. Make a list of exactly what drugs you are taking and give it to someone in your household or a nearby friend to use in case of emergency. If you were to faint or collapse, you would need someone to communicate for you with emergency personnel or doctors. This could prevent any dangerous interactions with drugs you may receive during emergency treatment.

Cutting costs on prescription drugs

It is possible to save money on prescriptions — you just have to know how. You will also need to do a little research on your own to find the best deals in your area. Here are some tips for putting your prescription drug dollars to good use.

Comparison shop. Neighborhood drugstores usually base their prices on what sells the most in their area. Prices may vary by as much as 25 percent, so it might be worth the drive to another pharmacy to get a better price.

Look for senior-citizen discounts. Many drugstores give good discounts to senior citizens.

Buy generic. Ask your doctor when he prescribes a drug if the generic form would be as effective for you. Generic drugs are usually cheaper than the brand-name forms, sometimes by as much as 50 percent. Some generic drugs may not be of the same quality as the brand-name equivalents, but some are just as good. You can ask your pharmacist to check on a generic drug in a publication called the *Orange Book*. He can tell you how much a particular generic varies, if any, from the equivalent brand-name drugs.

Buy in bulk. You can often save money by buying drugs you use all the time in larger quantities.

Ask for free samples. Find out if your doctor has any free samples of your new prescription so you can try it without investing any money. If there are no free samples, ask for a smaller prescription. That will allow you to be sure you tolerate the drug before you pay for a large prescription.

When you can't afford prescription drugs

If you know you don't have enough money to buy the drugs your doctor might prescribe for you, don't despair. There is a way to get help. Most major drug companies have an "Indigent Drug Program" to provide prescription drugs to people who can't afford them. You need to share this information with your doctor, since he is the one who must apply to the program for you.

Your doctor might already have a listing of these programs in the form of the *Directory of Prescription Drug Indigent Programs*. If not, he can get one by writing on office letterhead to:

Pharmaceutical Research & Manufacturers of America
1100 15th Street, N.W.
Washington, DC 20005
(800) 762-4636 or (800) 862-4110

If you prefer, you can call the drug companies yourself to find out how to apply for help. Here are six companies with indigent drug programs.

Hoechst Marion Roussel, Inc.
Patient Assistance Program
(800) 221-4025

Schering Plough Corporation
Commitment to Care
(800) 521-7157

Immunex Corporation
Patient Assistance Program
(800) 466-8639

Merck US Human Health
Patient Assistance Helpline
(800) 672-6372

TAP Pharmaceuticals
Care First Program
(800) 453-8438

ZENECA Pharmaceuticals
Assistant Programs
(800) 424-3727

How to use this chapter

Drugs are listed according to the condition they are intended to treat and conditions are listed alphabetically. For example, the drug section begins with drugs used to treat benign prostatic hyperplasia (BPH) and ends with drugs used to treat prostate cancer. Drugs are included for BPH, impotence, incontinence, pain, prostatitis and prostatodynia, and prostate cancer. Drugs are listed alphabetically within each section.

Each drug entry has several sections but not every entry includes all the sections. If one of the sections isn't used, it's because there was no information available on that aspect of the drug. Here is the basic layout for each listed drug:

Brand names: Here we list most of the common brand names of each drug. Sometimes you know your drug's brand name even though you don't know its generic name.

Drug type: You can use the drug type to look up more information from other sources.

Intended effect: This tells you what the medication is designed to treat and what action it will take in your body.

Side effects: This lists the side effects that may occur. They are listed from most common or frequent to least common and rare. Don't be concerned if there are a lot of side effects listed. Some side effects are natural, expected, and unavoidable. Most of them are unusual, unexpected, and infrequent. Some may depend on the size of the dose, and they will often go away if the dose is lowered. Remember, don't stop taking your medication or change the dosage without your doctor's approval.

Special warnings: This section will tell you when you should not take the drug, when you should take it with caution, and other important information. It is extremely important to notify your doctor if any of the warnings apply to you.

Possible food and drug interactions: This section tells you the foods and other drugs that may interact with the medicine you are taking.

Helpful hints: This section is included for most drugs and will give information on topics such as how and when to take the medication for best results.

When it comes to your health and the drugs your doctor prescribes to maintain it, you need to know as much as possible. Don't be afraid to take an active role in your health care by working closely with your doctor and pharmacist. It's your responsibility to know what drugs you are taking and how to use them appropriately.

We hope the information in this book will encourage you to communicate openly with your doctor and pharmacist to find the safest and most effective treatment for your prostate problem.

Benign prostatic hyperplasia (BPH)

Cyproterone
Brand name: Androcur (available in Canada)
Drug type: Antiandrogenic and antigonadatrophic
Intended effect: Blocks testosterone in addition to blocking the production of testosterone, which benign and malignant prostate cells need for growth. Suppresses hot flashes associated with a bilateral orchiectomy.
Side effects: Impotence, loss of sex drive, breast tenderness and enlargement, and a possibly higher risk of heart and blood vessel problems.

Special warnings:

- Some men taking this drug experience extreme tiredness. Either avoid driving or operating machinery or take extra precautions.

Possible food and drug interactions:

- Do not use alcohol while taking this drug.

Doxazosin
Brand name: Cardura
Drug type: Antihypertensive
Intended effect: Relaxes prostate muscles to improve urine flow.
Side effects: Dizziness, swelling, headache, tiredness, extremely low blood pressure, unusually fast heartbeat.

Special warnings:

- Don't drive or do any other potentially hazardous task for 24 hours after you take your first dose. Even after you've been taking the drug for a while, drive with caution. It may cause dizziness, lightheadedness, and palpitations at any time.

Possible food and drug interactions:

- If you take doxazosin with other blood pressure drugs, you're more likely to experience very low blood pressure and fainting.

- Alcohol can make your blood pressure drop even further while you're taking this drug.

Helpful hints:

- Taking the first dose at bedtime may help reduce the "first-dose" effect.

- Move slowly and carefully when you get up from a sitting or lying position.

Finasteride
Brand name: Proscar
Drug type: Antiandrogen
Intended effect: Reduces the size of the prostate.
Side effects: Impotence, decrease in the amount of semen you ejaculate, breast tenderness, skin rash.

Special warnings:

- Women who are pregnant or planning to become pregnant should not touch finasteride tablets or the semen of a man taking finasteride as it can cause birth defects in male fetuses.

Possible food and drug interactions:

- Talk with your doctor before taking over-the-counter medicines for colds, coughs, hay fever, asthma, or weight loss.

Helpful hint:

- Tablets may be crushed to make them easier to swallow.

Flutamide

Brand name: Eulexin

Drug type: Antiandrogen

Intended effect: Lowers output of testosterone to limit prostate growth and improve symptoms of BPH; treats prostate cancer that has spread to other parts of the body.

Side effects: Vomiting, diarrhea, nausea, hot flashes, impotence, breast enlargement, decreased sex drive, anemia, depression, low white blood cell count (lowered immunity), nervousness, anxiety, confusion, loss of appetite, fluid retention, high blood pressure.

Special warnings:

- Do not stop treatment without consulting your doctor.

- Periodic liver function tests should be performed.

Leuprolide acetate

Brand names: Lupron, Lupron Depot

Drug type: Androgen suppressor (LHRH agonist)

Intended effect: Suppresses the production of hormones including testosterone, which decreases the size of the prostate in men suffering from BPH; treats advanced cancer of the prostate.

Side effects: Hot flashes, impotence, headaches, pain, stomach upset, swelling, tiredness.

Special warnings:

- Early in treatment with leuprolide, testosterone levels may temporarily increase, resulting in a worsening of symptoms.

- Call your doctor as soon as possible if you experience chest pain or a fast or irregular heartbeat.

Prazosin

Brand name: Minipress

Drug type: Antihypertensive

Intended effect: Relaxes prostate muscles to improve urine flow.

Side effects: Dizziness, headaches, tiredness, sudden loss of consciousness, extremely low blood pressure, unusually fast heartbeat, nasal stuffiness.

Special warnings:

- You should take this drug cautiously if you're taking other blood pressure-lowering drugs or if you have poor liver function.

Possible food and drug interactions:

- If you take prazosin with other blood pressure drugs, you're more likely to experience very low blood pressure and fainting.

- Alcohol can make your blood pressure drop even further while you're taking this drug.

Helpful hints:

- Don't drive or do any other potentially hazardous task for 24 hours after you take your first dose. Even after you've been taking the drug for a while, drive with caution. It may cause dizziness, lightheadedness, and palpitations at any time.

- Taking the first dose at bedtime may help reduce the "first-dose" effect.

- Move slowly and carefully when you get up from a sitting or lying position.

Terazosin
Brand name: Hytrin
Drug type: Antihypertensive
Intended effect: Relaxes prostate muscles to improve urine flow.
Side effects: Dizziness, headaches, tiredness, nasal stuffiness, extremely low blood pressure, unusually fast heartbeat.

Special warnings:

- You should take this drug cautiously if you're taking other blood pressure-lowering drugs or if you have poor liver function.

Possible food and drug interactions:

- If you take terazosin with other blood pressure drugs, you're more likely to experience very low blood pressure and fainting.

- Alcohol can make your blood pressure drop even further while you're taking this drug.

Helpful hints:

- Don't drive or do any other potentially hazardous task for 24 hours after you take your first dose. Even after you've been taking the drug for a while, drive with caution. It may cause dizziness, lightheadedness, and palpitations at any time.

- Taking the first dose at bedtime may help reduce the "first-dose" effect.

- Move slowly and carefully when you get up from a sitting or lying position.

Impotence

Papaverine
Brand name: Pavabid
Drug type: Vasodilator
Intended effect: Expands blood vessels to increase blood flow.
Side effects: Nausea, dizziness, loss of appetite, constipation or diarrhea, headache, rash, sweating.

Special warnings:

- The effectiveness of this drug is lessened by smoking.

Helpful hints:

- Do not crush or break tablets.

- To avoid stomach upset, tablets may be taken with food, milk, or antacids.

- Move slowly and carefully when you get up from a sitting or lying position.

Phentolamine
Brand names: Regitine, Rogitine (in Canada)

Drug type: Alpha adrenergic blocker
Intended effect: Expands blood vessels to increase blood flow. Used in combination with papaverine as an injection into the penis to cause an erection.
Side effects: Tingling at the tip of the penis, low blood pressure, rapid or irregular heartbeat, weakness, dizziness, nausea, nasal stuffiness.

Special warnings:

- This injection should not be used by men who are not impotent. Improper use can result in permanent damage to the penis and impotence.

- Call your doctor if your erection lasts for more than four hours.

- Do not use more than once a day, more than two days in a row, or more than three times a week.

Helpful hints:

- Plan to have sex within two hours of the injection.

- Apply pressure to the injection site to prevent bruising.

- Massage the penis as directed by your doctor to help the drug spread over the entire penis.

Prostaglandin E1
Brand names: Alprostadil, Caverject
Drug type: Vasodilator
Intended effect: Expands blood vessels to increase blood flow. Used as an injection into the penis to cause an erection.
Side effects: Pain at injection site, burning sensation during erection.

Special warnings:

- This injection should not be used by men who are not impotent. Improper use can result in permanent damage to the penis and impotence.

- Call your doctor if your erection lasts for more than four hours.

- Do not use more than once a day, more than two days in a row, or more than three times a week.

Helpful hints:

- Plan to have sex within 30 minutes of the injection.

- Apply pressure to the injection site to prevent bruising.

- Massage the penis as directed by your doctor to help the drug spread over the entire penis.

Trazodone
Brand name: Desyrel
Drug type: Antidepressant
Intended effect: Improves mood and relieves anxiety and depression.
Side effects: Dizziness, dry mouth, nausea.

Special warnings:

- You shouldn't take trazodone when you are recovering from a heart attack. If you have heart disease, you should take this drug very cautiously. It can cause an irregular heartbeat.

- You should stop taking trazodone for as long as possible before surgery with general anesthesia.

Possible food and drug interactions:

- Since trazodone can cause low blood pressure, you may need a lower dose of your blood pressure-lowering drug.

- If you take trazodone along with any drug that depresses your nervous system, such as tranquilizers, alcohol, antihistamines, or muscle relaxers, the combination may seriously depress your nervous system.

- Trazodone may increase levels of the heart drug digoxin and the seizure drug phenytoin.

- Your doctor should monitor you carefully for side effects if you will be taking monoamine oxidase (MAO) inhibitors at the same time.

- Trazodone may cause increased bleeding if you take it while you are taking warfarin.

Helpful hints:

- Take trazadone after you eat a meal or snack. You will absorb it better and be less likely to feel dizzy and light-headed.

- As this drug can cause dizziness, you may want to take your largest dose at bedtime.

- Since this drug affects your central nervous system, you shouldn't drive a car or operate heavy machinery until you see how the medicine affects you.

Sildenafil citrate
Brand name: Viagra
Drug type: Phosphodiesterase type 5 inhibitors
Intended effect: Helps produce erections in men who are impotent.
Side effects: Headache, facial flushing, indigestion, nasal congestion, urinary tract infection, blurred vision, sensitivity to light, diarrhea, rash, dizziness.

Special warnings:

- Don't take Viagra if you are taking nitrates in any form, including the heart medicine nitroglycerin.

Helpful hint:

- You should take this drug about one hour before sexual activity.

Yohimbine
Brand names: Aphrodyne, Erex, Yocon, Yohimex
Drug type: Sympathicolytic
Intended effect: Helps produce erections in men who are impotent.
Side effects: Increased blood pressure, nervousness, irritability, rapid heart rate, headache, dizziness.

Special warnings:

- You shouldn't use this drug if you have a history of kidney disease, heart disease, or stomach or intestinal ulcers.

Possible food and drug interactions:

- Don't take this drug with antidepressants or other mood-altering drugs.

Helpful hint:

- It may take two to three weeks for this drug to begin to work.

Incontinence

Dicyclomine hydrochloride
Brand name: Bentyl
Drug type: Anticholinergic
Intended effect: Relieves cramps or spasms of the bladder.
Side effects: Headache, dizziness, drowsiness, confusion, palpitations, constipation.

Special warnings:

- This drug can make you overheated in hot weather. Watch for signs of heatstroke or fever.

Helpful hint:

- Since this drug may affect your central nervous system, you shouldn't drive a car or operate heavy machinery until you see how the medicine affects you.

Doxepin hydrochloride
Brand name: Sinequan, Triadapin
Drug type: Antidepressant
Intended effect: Relieves anxiety and depression by acting on the central nervous system.
Side effects: Headache, dry mouth, dizziness, nausea, diarrhea, ringing in the ears.

Special warnings:

- Since this drug may affect your central nervous system, you shouldn't drive a car or operate heavy machinery until you see how the medicine affects you.

- People with glaucoma should not take this drug.

Helpful hint:

- It may take two to three weeks for this drug to begin to work.

Flavoxate
Brand name: Urispas
Drug type: Antispasmodic
Intended effect: Relieves the symptoms of urinary incontinence and pain in the urinary tract.
Side effects: Dizziness, headache, difficulty concentrating, dry mouth, itching.

Special warnings:

- Men with enlarged prostates may have difficulty urinating while taking this drug.

- People with glaucoma should use this drug cautiously.

- Since this drug may affect your central nervous system, you shouldn't drive a car or operate heavy machinery until you see how the medicine affects you.

- This drug may make your eyes extra-sensitive to sunlight, so keep your sunglasses handy.

- Since this drug suppresses the sweating process, use it with caution in hot weather.

Helpful hint:

- Sucking on hard candy or ice chips may help relieve dry mouth.

Imipramine hydrochloride
Brand name: Janimine, Tofranil
Drug type: Antidepressant
Intended effect: Relieves anxiety and depression by acting on the central nervous system.

Side effects: Headache, dry mouth, dizziness, nausea, diarrhea, ringing in the ears.

Special warnings:

- Since this drug may affect your central nervous system, you shouldn't drive a car or operate heavy machinery until you see how the medicine affects you.

Helpful hints:

- This drug may make your skin extra-sensitive to sunlight, so protect your skin if you'll be outdoors in sunny weather.

- It may take two to three weeks for this drug to begin to work.

- Since imipramine has a sedative effect, you may want to take the largest dose in the afternoon or at bedtime.

Oxybutynin
Brand name: Ditropan
Drug type: Antispasmodic
Intended effect: Relieves the symptoms of urinary incontinence and pain in the urinary tract.
Side effects: Dizziness, drowsiness, rapid heartbeat, dry mouth, itching.

Special warnings:

- This drug may worsen heartbeat abnormalities.

- Since this drug may affect your central nervous system, you shouldn't drive a car or operate heavy machinery until you see how the medicine affects you.

- This drug may make your eyes extra-sensitive to sunlight, so keep your sunglasses handy.

- Since this drug suppresses the sweating process, use it with caution in hot weather.

Helpful hint:

- Sucking on hard candy or ice chips may help relieve dry mouth.

Pain

Mild to moderate pain

Ibuprofen
Brand names: Advil, IBU, IBU-TAB, Motrin
Drug type: Nonsteroidal anti-inflammatory drug (NSAID)
Intended effect: Relieves mild to moderate pain and reduces inflammation.
Side effects: Water retention, loss of appetite, ringing in the ears, dizziness, headache, stomach upset.

Special warnings:

- Don't use ibuprofen if you are allergic to aspirin or any NSAID.

- Take ibuprofen with caution if you have stomach ulcers, poor liver or kidney function, heart problems, high blood pressure, or blood-clotting disorders.

- Taking ibuprofen is more likely to cause kidney problems if you are elderly, if you take diuretics, or if you have lupus, heart failure, or poor liver or kidney function.

Possible food and drug interactions:

- Avoid alcohol while you're taking ibuprofen. Alcohol may increase your risk of internal bleeding.

- Ibuprofen may increase the effects of the cancer drug methotrexate.

- Ibuprofen may increase levels of the antipsychotic drug lithium.

- Ibuprofen may increase the effects of anticoagulants and the diuretic furosemide.

- Aspirin may decrease the anti-inflammatory effects of ibuprofen.

- If you need to stop corticosteroids while you're taking ibuprofen, be sure to withdraw slowly from the steroids instead of stopping suddenly.

Helpful hint:

- Take ibuprofen with food or a full glass of milk or water to prevent stomach irritation.

Flurbiprofen
Brand names: Ansaid, Froben
Drug type: Nonsteroidal anti-inflammatory drug (NSAID)
Intended effect: Relieves mild to moderate pain and reduces inflammation.
Side effects: Stomach cramps, dizziness, drowsiness, heartburn, nausea, headache.

Special warnings:

- Don't use flurbiprofen if you are allergic to aspirin or any NSAID.

- Take flurbiprofen with caution if you have stomach ulcers, poor heart function, high blood pressure, or blood-clotting disorders.

- Taking flurbiprofen is more likely to cause kidney problems if you are elderly; if you take diuretics; or if you have lupus, heart failure, or poor liver or kidney function.

Possible food and drug interactions:

- Avoid alcohol and aspirin while taking flurbiprofen.

- Flurbiprofen may prolong bleeding time if used at the same time as anticoagulants.

- Flurbiprofen may decrease the effects of beta-blockers and diuretics.

Helpful hints:

- Take flurbiprofen with food or a full glass of milk or water to prevent stomach irritation.

- Don't drive a car or operate heavy machinery until you are sure the medicine isn't making you drowsy or less than alert.

Moderate pain

Codeine
Brand names: Codeine, Paveral (in Canada)
Drug type: Narcotic analgesic
Intended effect: Relieves moderate pain by acting on the central nervous system.
Side effects: Nausea, vomiting, dry mouth, dizziness, drowsiness.

Special warnings:

- Since this drug can make you drowsy, you shouldn't drive a car or operate heavy machinery until you see how the medicine affects you.

- Long-term use of narcotics can result in dependence and withdrawal symptoms when you stop taking the drug. Tell your doctor if you have a history of drug or alcohol abuse.

- Do not drink alcohol while taking codeine.

Helpful hints:

- Move slowly and carefully when you get up from a sitting or lying position.

- Sucking on hard candy or ice chips may help relieve dry mouth.

Oxycodone
Brand name: Roxicodone, Percodan
Drug type: Narcotic analgesic
Intended effect: Relieves moderate pain by acting on the central nervous system.
Side effects: Nausea, vomiting, dry mouth, dizziness, drowsiness.

Special warnings:

- Since this drug can make you drowsy, you shouldn't drive a car or operate heavy machinery until you see how the medicine affects you.

- Long-term use of narcotics can result in dependence and withdrawal symptoms when you stop taking the drug.

- Do not drink alcohol while taking this drug.

Helpful hints:

- Move slowly and carefully when you get up from a sitting or lying position.

- Sucking on hard candy or ice chips may help relieve dry mouth.

Severe pain

Morphine
Brand names: Astramorph, Duramorph, Kadian, MS Contin, MSIR
Drug type: Narcotic analgesic
Intended effect: Relieves severe pain by acting on the central nervous system.
Side effects: Nausea, vomiting, dry mouth, dizziness, drowsiness.

Special warnings:

- Since this drug can make you drowsy, you shouldn't drive a car or operate heavy machinery until you see how the medicine affects you.

- Long-term use of narcotics can result in dependence and withdrawal symptoms when you stop taking the drug.

- Do not drink alcohol while taking morphine.

Helpful hints:

- Move slowly and carefully when you get up from a sitting or lying position.

- Sucking on hard candy or ice chips may help relieve dry mouth.

Methadone
Brand name: Dolophine
Drug type: Narcotic analgesic
Intended effect: Relieves severe pain by acting on the central nervous system.
Side effects: Nausea, vomiting, dry mouth, dizziness, drowsiness.

Special warnings:

- Since this drug can make you drowsy, you shouldn't drive a car or operate heavy machinery until you see how the medicine affects you.

- Long-term use of narcotics can result in dependence and withdrawal symptoms when you stop taking the drug.

- Do not drink alcohol while taking methadone.

Helpful hints:

- Move slowly and carefully when you get up from a sitting or lying position.

- Sucking on hard candy or ice chips may help relieve dry mouth.

Fentanyl
Brand name: Sublimaze
Drug type: Narcotic analgesic
Intended effect: Relieves severe pain by acting on the central nervous system.
Side effects: Nausea, vomiting, dizziness, drowsiness.

Special warnings:

- Since this drug can make you drowsy, you shouldn't drive a car or operate heavy machinery until you see how the medicine affects you.

- Long-term use of narcotics can result in dependence and withdrawal symptoms when you stop taking the drug.

- Do not drink alcohol while taking fentanyl.

Helpful hint:

- Move slowly and carefully when you get up from a sitting or lying position.

Chronic pain

Desipramine
Brand names: Norpramin, Pertofrane

Drug type: Tricyclic antidepressant
Intended effect: Relieves chronic pain and mental depression.
Side effects: Headache, dizziness, drowsiness, dry mouth.

Special warnings:

- Since this drug can make you drowsy, you shouldn't drive a car or operate heavy machinery until you see how the medicine affects you.

- Do not drink alcohol while taking desipramine.

Helpful hints:

- This drug may make your skin extra-sensitive to sunlight, so protect your skin if you'll be outdoors in sunny weather.

- Move slowly and carefully when you get up from a sitting or lying position.

- Sucking on hard candy or ice chips may help relieve dry mouth.

Imipramine
Brand names: Norfranil, Tipramine, Tofranil
Drug type: Tricyclic antidepressant, bladder antispasmodic
Intended effect: Relieves chronic pain, bladder spasms, and mental depression.
Side effects: Headache, dizziness, drowsiness, dry mouth.

Special warnings:

- Since this drug can make you drowsy, you shouldn't drive a car or operate heavy machinery until you see how the medicine affects you.

- Do not drink alcohol while taking imipramine.

Helpful hints:

- This drug may make your skin extra-sensitive to sunlight, so protect your skin if you'll be outdoors in sunny weather.

- Move slowly and carefully when you get up from a sitting or lying position.

- Sucking on hard candy or ice chips may help relieve dry mouth.

Nortriptyline
Brand name: Pamelor
Drug type: Tricyclic antidepressant
Intended effect: Relieves chronic pain and mental depression.
Side effects: Headache, dizziness, drowsiness, dry mouth.

Special warnings:

- Since this drug can make you drowsy, you shouldn't drive a car or operate heavy machinery until you see how the medicine affects you.

- Do not drink alcohol while taking nortriptyline.

Helpful hints:

- This drug may make your skin extra-sensitive to sunlight, so protect your skin if you'll be outdoors in sunny weather.

- Move slowly and carefully when you get up from a sitting or lying position.

- Sucking on hard candy or ice chips may help relieve dry mouth.

Prostatitis and prostatodynia

Allopurinol
Brand names: Zyloprim, Lopurin
Drug type: Antigout agent
Intended effect: Decreases the amount of uric acid produced by the body.
Side effects: Nausea, headache, drowsiness, diarrhea, skin rash, gout attack.

Special warnings:

- Call your doctor at the first sign of rash or allergic reaction. Taking this drug along with ampicillin or amoxicillin increases the chances of skin rash.

Possible food and drug interactions:

- Allopurinol may increase the effects of anticoagulants.

- Allopurinol may increase the effects of azathioprine or mer-captopurine.

Helpful hints:

- Since this drug can make you drowsy, you shouldn't drive a car or operate heavy machinery until you see how the medicine affects you.

- Drink at least 10 cups of water a day while taking allopurinol to help prevent kidney stones from forming.

Ampicillin
Brand names: Ampicin, Omnipen
Drug type: Antibiotic
Intended effect: Kills bacteria that are causing infection.
Side effects: Mild rash, stomach upset, diarrhea.

Special warnings:

- This drug should not be used by people allergic to penicillin or cephalosporin antibiotics.

- People with diabetes may have false-positive sugar tests.

- Dangerous sensitivity reactions can occur, causing symptoms such as fainting, shortness of breath, fever, red skin rash, hives, or swelling of the face. Call your doctor at the first sign of rash or allergic reaction.

Possible food and drug interactions:

- Probenecid may increase levels of ampicillin in the blood.

- Taking this drug along with allopurinol increases the chances of skin rash.

Helpful hint:

- To improve absorption of the drug, take it on an empty stomach — at least one hour before or two hours after a meal.

Amoxicillin

Brand name: Amoxil
Drug type: Antibiotic
Intended effect: Kills bacteria that are causing infection.
Side effects: Mild rash, stomach upset, diarrhea.

Special warnings:

- This drug should not be used by people allergic to penicillin or cephalosporin antibiotics.

- People with diabetes may have false-positive sugar tests.

- Call your doctor immediately if fainting, shortness of breath, fever, red skin rash, hives, or swelling of the face occurs, since they could indicate an allergic reaction.

Possible food and drug interactions:

- Taking this drug along with allopurinol increases the chances of skin rash.

Helpful hints:

- Take all of your prescription, even after your symptoms go away.

- Most penicillins shouldn't be taken with food, but you can take amoxicillin with food to help prevent upset stomach.

Carbenicillin

Brand name: Geocillin
Drug type: Antibiotic
Intended effect: Kills bacteria that are causing infection.
Side effects: Nausea, bad taste in the mouth, diarrhea, gas, and swelling of the tongue.

Special warnings:

- Do not use this drug if you are allergic to penicillin, as severe allergic reaction can occur.

- Long-term use may lead to development of resistant bacteria in the body.

- People with kidney problems, liver problems, and blood disorders should take this drug with caution.

Possible food and drug interactions:

- Probenecid may increase levels of carbenicillin in the blood.

Helpful hint:

- To improve absorption of carbenicillin, take it on an empty stomach — at least one hour before or two hours after a meal.

Cephalexin
Brand names: C-Lexin, Keflex, Keftab, Novo-Lexin
Drug type: Antimicrobial
Intended effect: Kills bacteria that are causing infection. Sometimes injections of cephalexin are given before surgery to prevent infection.
Side effects: Diarrhea, stomach cramps, fever, bruising, sore tongue.

Special warnings:

- People with diabetes may have false-positive sugar tests.

Possible food and drug interactions:

- Avoid alcohol while you're taking cephalexin and for several days afterward.

Ciprofloxacin
Brand name: Cipro
Drug type: Antimicrobial
Intended effect: Kills bacteria that are causing infection.
Side effects: Stomach upset, headache, restlessness, rash.

Special warnings:

- Do not use if you have any allergies to drugs in the quinolone class.

- Dangerous sensitivity reactions can occur, causing symptoms such as swelling of the face or throat, difficult breathing (such as an asthma attack), itching, hives, tingling, or loss of consciousness. Call your doctor at the first sign of rash or allergic reaction.

- People with any condition that increases the risk of seizures should use ciprofloxacin with caution.

- The dose may need to be adjusted for people with poor kidney function.

- Kidney and liver function tests and certain blood tests should be done periodically while taking this drug.

Possible food and drug interactions:

- Ciprofloxacin may increase the effects of caffeine, the asthma drug theophylline, and the anticoagulant warfarin.

- Antacids, some iron pills, and multivitamins containing zinc may decrease absorption of this drug.

- Probenecid, a drug used to decrease uric acid production, may increase levels of ciprofloxacin in the blood.

Helpful hints:

- Although this drug may be taken with food, it is best taken two hours after you eat.

- Drink plenty of fluids while taking this drug.

- Use caution while driving. Ciprofloxacin may cause dizziness or lightheadedness.

- This drug may make your skin extra-sensitive to sunlight, so protect your skin if you'll be outdoors in sunny weather.

Clindamycin
Brand name: Cleocin
Drug type: Antimicrobial
Intended effect: Kills bacteria that are causing infection.
Side effects: Stomach pain, nausea, diarrhea, rash, itching, jaundice (yellow eyes and skin).

Special warnings:

- People with kidney disease, liver disease, or a history of intestinal diseases, such as colitis, should not use this drug. Call your doctor immediately if severe diarrhea develops.

Possible food and drug interactions:

- This drug may increase the effect of muscle relaxers.

Helpful hint:

- Take this drug with a glass of water to avoid irritating your esophagus.

Doxazosin

Brand name: Cardura
Drug type: Alpha adrenergic blocker
Intended effect: Relieves spasms of the bladder neck, urethral sphincter, and pelvic floor.
Side effects: Dizziness, swelling, tiredness, extremely low blood pressure, unusually fast heartbeat.

Possible food and drug interactions:

- If you take doxazosin with other blood pressure drugs, you're more likely to experience very low blood pressure and fainting.

- Alcohol can make your blood pressure drop even further while you're taking this drug.

Helpful hints:

- Don't drive or do any other potentially hazardous task for 24 hours after you take your first dose. Even after you've been taking the drug for a while, drive with caution. It may cause dizziness, lightheadedness, and palpitations at any time.

- Taking the first dose at bedtime may help reduce the "first-dose" effect.

- Move slowly and carefully when you get up from a sitting or lying position.

Doxycycline hyclate

Brand names: Doryx, Vibramycin, Vibra-Tabs
Drug type: Antimicrobial
Intended effect: Treats prostatitis caused by chlamydia infections.
Side effects: Stomach upset, loss of appetite, sore throat or hoarseness, inflammation of the mouth or tongue, difficulty swallowing, rash, light sensitivity, blue-gray discoloration of the skin, liver or kidney problems, hives, fluid retention, fever, joint pain, worsening of lupus.

Special warnings:

- Do not use this drug if you are allergic to tetracycline antibiotics.

- Discontinue use if allergic skin reaction appears after exposure to sunlight.

- If you have kidney problems, tetracyclines can accumulate to toxic levels in your body.

Possible food and drug interactions:

- This drug may increase the levels or effects of anticoagulants, and it may interfere with the actions of penicillin antibiotics.

- Antacids and iron-containing products may reduce the absorption of this drug.

Helpful hints:

- Take with food or milk to avoid stomach irritation. Make sure you wash down the drug with plenty of liquid to prevent ulcers and irritation of your esophagus and throat, especially if you will be lying down afterward.

- This drug may make your skin extra-sensitive to sunlight, so protect your skin if you'll be outdoors in sunny weather.

Enoxacin

Brand name: Penetrex
Drug type: Fluoroquinolone antimicrobial
Intended effect: Kills bacteria that cause urinary tract infections.
Side effects: Dizziness, nausea, vomiting, stomach pain, headache.

Special warnings:

- Tell your doctor if you have ever had a seizure before taking enoxacin.

Possible food and drug interactions:

- Enoxacin can increase the effects of the anticoagulant warfarin, raising the risk of bleeding.

- Don't drink caffeinated beverages such as coffee, tea, or cola; eat foods with caffeine such as chocolate; or take medicines that contain caffeine while taking enoxacin.

- Take antacids, vitamins, or any products containing iron or zinc eight hours before or two hours after taking enoxacin.

Helpful hints:

- Drink plenty of fluids while taking enoxacin.

- Enoxacin should be taken on an empty stomach.

- You shouldn't drive a car or operate heavy machinery until you are sure this medicine isn't making you drowsy or less than alert.

- This drug may make your skin extra-sensitive to sunlight, so protect your skin if you'll be outdoors in sunny weather.

Erythromycin
Brand names: E-mycin, ERYC, Ery-Tab, PCE Dispertab
Drug type: Antimicrobial
Intended effect: Kills bacteria that are causing infection.
Side effects: Nausea, loss of appetite, diarrhea, stomach cramps and discomfort, itching, skin rash, irregular heartbeat.

Special warnings:

- People with liver disease should not take this drug.

Possible food and drug interactions:

- This drug may cause rhabdomyolysis (a disease that destroys muscle tissue) in people taking the cholesterol-reducer lovastatin.

- This drug may increase the levels or effects of anticoagulants, the seizure drug carbamazepine, the heart drug digoxin, the migraine drug ergotamine, the asthma drug theophylline, and the insomnia drug triazolam.

- Taking terfenadine and erythromycin together can cause life-threatening heart-rhythm disturbances.

Helpful hints:

- The effectiveness of erythromycin is decreased in some people when they take it with food. If it upsets your stomach, take it with food. If it doesn't, take it on an empty stomach — one hour before or two hours after meals.

- Take each dose at evenly spaced intervals throughout the day with at least six ounces of fluids.

Gentamicin
Brand names: Garamycin, G-Mycin, Jenamicin, Cidomycin (in Canada)
Drug type: Aminoglycoside
Intended effect: Kills bacteria that are causing serious infection.
Side effects: Hearing loss, ringing in the ears, change in urinary habits, dizziness, headache.

Special warnings:

- High doses of this drug over long periods can cause kidney damage and hearing loss.

- Tell your doctor if you are allergic to any foods or preservatives (such as sulfites) or have any of the following medical conditions: kidney disease, Parkinson's disease, hearing loss or balance problems, or myasthenia gravis.

Helpful hint:

- This drug is only given intravenously (injected into a vein).

Ketoconazole
Brand name: Nizoral
Drug type: Antifungal

Intended effect: Treats prostatitis caused by a yeast infection.
Side effects: Nausea, itching, stomach pain.

Special warnings:

- Liver functions should be tested before treatment begins and should be carefully monitored during treatment, especially in people with a history of liver disease.

- This drug should be used with caution by men who have prostate cancer.

Possible food and drug interactions:

- Do not take ketoconazole with the allergy drug terfenadine because it may cause a dangerously rapid heartbeat.

- Taking this drug with the antihistamine astemizole may cause heartbeat irregularities.

- Antacids should be taken two hours after this drug because they reduce absorption.

- Effects of this drug may be decreased by anticholinergics, histamine blockers, and the tuberculosis drug rifampin.

- This drug may increase levels or effects of corticosteroids, anticoagulants, and the immunosuppressant cyclosporine.

- If taken with the antifungal drug miconazole, this drug may cause very low blood sugar.

Helpful hints:

- You shouldn't drive a car or operate heavy machinery until you are sure this medicine isn't making you drowsy, dizzy, or less than alert.

- Take your medicine with food to help prevent nausea. Nausea should go away after you've been taking the drug for a while.

- This drug may make your skin extra-sensitive to sunlight, so protect your skin if you'll be outdoors in sunny weather.

Levofloxacin

Brand name: Levaquin
Drug type: Fluoroquinolone
Intended effect: Kills bacteria that are causing urinary tract infections and prostatitis.
Side effects: Nausea, diarrhea, headache, and constipation.

Possible food and drug interactions:

- Take levofloxacin two hours before or two hours after taking antacids, vitamins, or mineral supplements.

Helpful hint:

- This drug may make your skin extra-sensitive to sunlight, so protect your skin if you'll be outdoors in sunny weather.

Lomefloxacin

Brand name: Maxaquin
Drug type: Fluoroquinolone
Intended effect: Kills bacteria that are causing serious infection and prevents infections after transurethral procedures.
Side effects: Dizziness, headache, drowsiness, nausea, diarrhea, cough, itching, skin rash.
Possible food and drug interactions:

- Wait at least four hours after taking lomefloxacin before taking any antacids that contain aluminum or magnesium.

- Probenecid slows the breakdown of lomefloxacin in the body, which can allow toxic levels to accumulate.

Helpful hints:

- This drug may make your skin extra-sensitive to sunlight, so protect your skin if you'll be outdoors in sunny weather.

- You shouldn't drive a car or operate heavy machinery until you are sure this medicine isn't making you drowsy, dizzy, or less than alert.

Minocycline
Brand name: Minocin
Drug type: Tetracycline antimicrobial
Intended effect: Kills bacteria that are causing infection.
Side effects: Stomach pain, vomiting, nausea, skin rash, sore tongue, dizziness, faintness.

Possible food and drug interactions:

- Take minocycline one hour before or two hours after eating any dairy products or taking any antacids that contain aluminum or magnesium.

Helpful hints:

- This drug may make your skin extra-sensitive to sunlight, so protect your skin if you'll be outdoors in sunny weather.

- You shouldn't drive a car or operate heavy machinery until you are sure this medicine isn't making you drowsy, dizzy, or less than alert.

Nitrofurantoin
Brand names: Furadantin, Macrobid, Macrodantin
Drug type: Antimicrobial
Intended effect: Kills bacteria that are causing infection.
Side effects: Headache, dizziness, drowsiness, diarrhea, nausea, vomiting, itching, difficulty breathing.

Special warnings:

- In people with G6PD deficiency, this drug may cause anemia.

- People with diabetes may have false-positive sugar tests.

Possible food and drug interactions:

- Side effects may be increased if nitrofurantoin is taken with probenecid.

Helpful hint:

- Take this drug with food or milk to absorb it better and lessen stomach upset.

Norfloxacin

Brand name: Noroxin
Drug type: Antibacterial
Intended effect: Relieves inflammation of the prostate.
Side effects: Dizziness, stomach upset, loss of appetite, tiredness, rash, sweating.

Special warnings:

- This drug should not be taken if you have allergies to fluoroquinolones or quinolone antibacterials or are under 18 years of age.

- If you have any disorders of the central nervous system, such as epilepsy, which may increase your risk of seizures, you should use this drug with caution.

- Kidney and liver function should be checked and blood tests done periodically while you are taking this drug.

Possible food and drug interactions:

- Take antacids, vitamins, or any products containing iron or zinc four hours before or two hours after taking norfloxacin.

- This drug may increase the effects of caffeine, the anticoagulant warfarin, the immunosuppressant cyclosporine, and the asthma drug theophylline.

- Levels of this drug may be increased by probenecid, a drug used to treat gout.

- Effects of this drug may be decreased by the antibacterial drug nitrofurantoin.

Helpful hints:

- Take on an empty stomach — one hour before or two hours after meals.

- Drink plenty of fluids while you are taking this drug.

- This drug may make your skin extra-sensitive to sunlight, so protect your skin if you'll be outdoors in sunny weather.

- You shouldn't drive a car or operate heavy machinery until you are sure this medicine isn't making you drowsy, dizzy, or less than alert.

Nystatin
Brand name: Nystatin
Drug type: Antifungal
Intended effect: To treat prostatitis caused by a yeast infection.
Side effects: Stomach upset, rash, diarrhea.

Ofloxacin
Brand name: Floxin
Drug type: Quinolone antimicrobial
Intended effect: Kills bacteria that are causing inflammation of the prostate.
Side effects: Headache, stomach upset, insomnia, itching, rash, altered sense of taste, chest pain, dry mouth, nervousness, fever, sore throat, loss of appetite, gas, tiredness, constipation.

Special warnings:

- This drug should not be taken by people with allergies to fluoroquinolones or quinolone medication. Serious, sometimes fatal, allergic reactions can occur, causing symptoms such as swelling of the face or throat, difficulty breathing, itching, hives, tingling, or loss of consciousness.

- If you have any disorders of the central nervous system, such as epilepsy, which may increase the risk of seizures, you should use this drug with caution. People with diabetes or poor kidney or liver function should also use it with caution.

- Blood glucose levels and liver and kidney functions should be checked periodically. If low blood sugar occurs in diabetics, stop taking the drug and call your doctor.

Possible food and drug interactions:

- This drug may increase the effects of the anticoagulant warfarin and the immunosuppressant cyclosporine.

- Levels or effects of ofloxacin may be decreased by the antibacterial drug nitrofurantoin.

- Take antacids, vitamins, or any products containing iron or zinc four hours before or two hours after taking ofloxacin.

- If taken with nonsteroidal anti-inflammatory drugs (NSAIDs), ofloxacin may increase the risk of seizure.

Helpful hints:

- Take one hour before or two hours after meals.

- Sensitivity to light may occur even when sunscreens or sunblocks are used and may persist after treatment is stopped.

- You shouldn't drive a car or operate heavy machinery until you are sure this medicine isn't making you drowsy or less than alert.

Prazosin
Brand name: Minipress
Drug type: Alpha adrenergic blocker
Intended effect: Relieves spasms of the bladder neck, urethral sphincter, and pelvic floor.
Side effects: Dizziness, headaches, tiredness, sudden loss of consciousness, extremely low blood pressure, unusually fast heartbeat, nasal stuffiness.

Special warnings:

- You should take this drug cautiously if you're taking other blood pressure-lowering drugs or if you have poor liver function.

Possible food and drug interactions:

- If you take prazosin with other blood pressure drugs, you're more likely to experience very low blood pressure and fainting.

- Alcohol can make your blood pressure drop even further while you're taking this drug.

Helpful hints:

- Don't drive or do any other potentially hazardous task for 24 hours after you take your first dose. Even after you've been taking the drug for a while, drive with caution. It may cause dizziness, lightheadedness, and palpitations at any time.

- Taking the first dose at bedtime may help reduce the "first-dose" effect.

- Move slowly and carefully when you get up from a sitting or lying position.

Penicillin G procaine

Brand names: Wycillin, Ayercillin (in Canada)
Drug type: Antibiotic
Intended effect: Kills bacteria that are causing infection.
Side effects: Dizziness, chills, fever, skin rash, shortness of breath.

Special warnings:

- If diarrhea develops while you are taking this drug, call your doctor before you take any diarrhea medicine.

- People with diabetes may have false-positive sugar tests.

Helpful hint:

- If you are taking the pill form of penicillin G, don't drink acidic fruit juices (such as orange and grapefruit) for one hour after taking this drug.

Tetracycline

Brand names: Achromycin, Terramycin
Drug type: Antibiotic
Intended effect: Treats prostatitis caused by chlamydia infections.
Side effects: Light sensitivity, difficulty swallowing, loss of appetite, stomach upset, swelling of the tongue, rash, itching, fluid retention, lupus, ringing in the ears, abnormal liver function.

Special warnings:

- Tetracycline may accumulate to toxic levels in people with kidney problems.

Possible food and drug interactions:

- Tetracycline may increase the effect of anticoagulants.

- This drug may decrease the effects of the antibiotic penicillin.

- Levels of this drug may be decreased by antacids.

Helpful hints:

- Take on an empty stomach, with a full glass of water, one hour before or two hours after meals.

- Liver tests should be performed regularly during treatment.

Tobramycin
Brand name: Nebcin
Drug type: Aminoglycoside antibiotic
Intended effect: Kills bacteria that are causing serious infections.
Side effects: Headache, ringing in the ears, dizziness, nausea, loss of appetite, skin rash.

Special warnings:

- High doses of this drug over long periods can cause kidney damage and hearing loss.

- Tell your doctor if you are allergic to any foods or preservatives (such as sulfites) or have any of the following medical conditions: kidney disease, Parkinson's disease, hearing loss or balance problems, or myasthenia gravis.

Helpful hints:

- This drug is only given intravenously (injected into a vein).

- Drink plenty of fluids while taking this drug.

Trimethoprim/sulfamethoxazole
Brand names: Bactrim, Bactrim DS, Septra, Septra DS
Drug type: Sulfonamide antibacterial
Intended effect: Kills bacteria that are causing infection.
Side effects: Stomach upset, loss of appetite, stomach pain, swelling and redness of mouth or tongue, inflammation of the intestines and colon, headache, depression, insomnia, drowsiness, convulsions, hallucinations, ringing in the ears, hearing loss, dizziness, lack of muscle coordination, joint pain, fever, chills, hair loss, sensitivity to sunlight.

Special warnings:

- People with poor liver or kidney function, asthma, folate deficiency, malnutrition, or G6PD deficiency should use this drug with caution. This drug may cause destruction of red blood cells in people with G6PD.

- Blood and urine should be tested regularly during treatment.

Possible food and drug interactions:

- This drug may increase levels or effects of the seizure drug phenytoin and the anticoagulant warfarin. It may also increase levels of the cancer drug methotrexate to toxic levels.

- This drug may cause blood disorders in elderly people who are taking diuretics.

Helpful hints:

- To help prevent kidney disorders, drink at least four to six glasses of water every day while taking this drug.

- Take with food or milk if this drug upsets your stomach. If it doesn't upset your stomach, take it one hour before or two hours after a meal.

- This drug may make your skin extra-sensitive to sunlight, so protect your skin if you'll be outdoors in sunny weather.

Prostate cancer

Aminoglutethimide
Brand name: Cytadren
Drug type: Antiandrogen, antineoplastic
Intended effect: Stops the adrenal glands from producing testosterone.
Side effects: Nausea, loss of appetite, headache, dizziness, drowsiness.

Special warnings:

- Don't drive or do any other potentially hazardous task for 24 hours after you take your first dose. Even after you've been taking the drug for a while, drive with caution. It may cause dizziness, lightheadedness, and palpitations at any time.

- Let your doctor know if you have recently been exposed to chickenpox or if you've had shingles.

Possible food and drug interactions:

- Don't drink alcohol while taking this drug.

Helpful hint:

- Move slowly and carefully when you get up from a sitting or lying position.

Bicalutamide
Brand name: Casodex
Drug type: Antiandrogen
Intended effect: Stops the production of androgens in the body.
Side effects: Constipation, diarrhea, hot flashes, breast pain, breast enlargement.

Cyproterone
Brand name: Androcur (available in Canada)
Drug type: Antiandrogenic and antigonadatrophic
Intended effect: Blocks testosterone in addition to blocking the production of testosterone, which benign and malignant prostate cells need for growth. Suppresses hot flashes associated with a bilateral orchiectomy.
Side effects: Impotence, loss of sex drive, breast tenderness and enlargement, and a possibly higher risk of heart and blood vessel problems.

Special warnings:

- Some men taking this drug experience extreme tiredness. Either avoid driving or operating machinery or take extra precautions.

Possible food and drug interactions:

- Do not use alcohol while taking this drug.

Diethylstilbestrol

Brand name: DES
Drug type: Estrogen
Intended effect: Treats the symptoms of advanced prostate cancer.
Side effects: Vomiting, nausea, breast enlargement, impotence, headache, fluid retention.

Special warnings:

- Men who take diethylstilbestrol for a long time increase their risk of heart disease.

- This drug should be used cautiously in men with migraines, epilepsy, kidney disease, and heart disease.

Helpful hint:

- This drug can be taken with or after meals to avoid stomach upset.

Estradiol

Brand name: Estrace
Drug type: Systemic estrogen
Intended effect: Treats inoperable prostate cancer.
Side effects: Breast enlargement, loss of sex drive, hot flashes, impotence, stomach upset, headache, dizziness, depression, rash, joint pain, light sensitivity, increased risk of blood clots.

Special warnings:

- Smoking increases your risk of developing serious side effects, such as stroke, heart attacks, and blood clots.

- If you experience any signs of a blood clot — shortness of breath, pain in your chest or legs, a severe headache, dizziness, or faintness — call your doctor immediately.

Possible food and drug interactions:

- Be sure to tell your doctor if you are taking phenobarbital, warfarin, phenytoin, rifampin, amitriptyline, or imipramine.

Helpful hints:

- Take this drug after meals or with a snack if you experience nausea.

- Wear a sunscreen when you go outdoors if your skin burns more easily.

Flutamide
Brand name: Eulexin
Drug type: Antiandrogen
Intended effect: Lowers output of testosterone to limit prostate growth and improve symptoms of BPH; treats prostate cancer that has spread to other parts of the body.
Side effects: Vomiting, diarrhea, nausea, hot flashes, impotence, breast enlargement, decreased sex drive, anemia, depression, low white blood cell count (lowered immunity), nervousness, anxiety, confusion, loss of appetite, fluid retention, high blood pressure.

Special warnings:

- Do not stop treatment without consulting your doctor.

- Periodic liver function tests should be performed.

Goserelin acetate
Brand name: Zoladex
Drug type: Androgen suppressor (LHRH agonist)
Intended effect: Treats the symptoms of advanced prostate cancer by blocking the production of testosterone.
Side effects: Tiredness, dizziness, headache, nausea, irregular heartbeat, hot flashes, breast enlargement.

Special warnings:

- Early in treatment with goserelin, testosterone levels may temporarily increase, resulting in a worsening of symptoms.

Leuprolide acetate
Brand names: Lupron, Lupron Depot
Drug type: Androgen suppressor (LHRH agonist)

Intended effect: Treats the symptoms of advanced prostate cancer by blocking the production of testosterone.
Side effects: Hot flashes, impotence, headaches, pain, stomach upset, swelling, tiredness.

Special warnings:

- Early in treatment with leuprolide, testosterone levels may temporarily increase, resulting in a worsening of symptoms.

- Call your doctor as soon as possible if you experience chest pain or a fast or irregular heartbeat.

Megestrol
Brand name: Megace
Drug type: Antiandrogen; progesterone agent
Intended effect: Suppresses prostate cancer especially if used with another agent such as estrogen. Also suppresses hot flashes associated with bilateral orchiectomy or anti-androgen therapy.
Side effects: Weight gain

Special warnings:

- Men with a history of blood clots should use this drug with caution.

Mitoxantrone
Brand name: Novantrone
Drug type: Antineoplastic
Intended effect: Relieves the pain associated with advanced prostate cancer.
Side effects: Nausea, vomiting, diarrhea, blue-green tint to urine or whites of eyes, hair loss, skin rash, headache, tiredness.

Special warnings:

- Call your doctor as soon as possible if you experience chest pain, difficulty breathing, or a fast or irregular heartbeat.

- This drug may cause you to bleed more than usual from a cut or injury.

Helpful hints:

- Brush and floss your teeth gently to avoid gum bleeding.

- You may be more likely to catch colds and other illnesses while taking mitoxantrone, so avoid people who are sick and wash your hands frequently.

Glossary

A

Acid phosphatase — An enzyme produced only in the prostate. High levels may indicate the spread of prostate cancer.

Acute bacterial prostatitis — A rare condition that involves sudden, sometimes severe, inflammation or infection of the prostate. Symptoms include fever and burning during urination. Generally responds quickly to antibiotics.

Acute urinary retention — Condition that requires immediate medical attention, occurring when the urethra is squeezed so tightly by the prostate that it becomes impossible to urinate. Things that can trigger urinary retention include delaying urination, urinary tract infection, alcohol intake, antidepressants, decongestants, tranquilizers, cold temperatures, and being still for long periods of time.

Adrenal glands — Two endocrine organs lying immediately above the kidney. They produce epinephrine, norepinephrine, and a variety of steroid hormones, including testosterone.

Alpha blockers — The same medicine used to treat high blood pressure that can relieve BPH and incontinence symptoms in men with an enlarged prostate. Relaxes the smooth muscles that are squeezing the urethra, making it harder for urine to get through.

Androgens — Male hormones.

Androgen-dependent cells — Prostate cancer cells that need androgen hormones to grow. Hormone therapy will control these kinds of cells.

Androgen-independent cells — Prostate cancer cells that don't need androgen hormones to grow. No treatments, including hormone therapy, will control these kinds of cells.

Antiandrogens — Drugs that block testosterone from binding with receptors in the prostate.

Artificial sphincter — A three-part device that is surgically implanted near the bladder to control incontinence.

Asymptomatic prostatitis — A new category in the classification of prostatitis. This type of prostatitis causes no symptoms. It is often diagnosed during a test for prostate cancer.

Atherosclerosis — A condition in which fatty deposits build up in your blood vessels, restricting blood flow. A common cause of impotence, especially in older men.

B

Balloon dilation — A new version of the old technique of prostate dilation used for treating BPH. A catheter with a balloon at the end is inserted through the urethra and into the prostatic urethra. The balloon is then inflated to stretch the urethra where narrowed by the prostate. This treatment is not very effective and is not used much anymore.

Benign prostatic hyperplasia (BPH) — A noncancerous enlargement of the prostate gland that commonly affects half the men over age 60. Extra tissue grows inside the prostate and presses on the urethra. This prevents your bladder from being emptied completely and leads to annoying symptoms like dribbling, a slow stream, and frequent urination.

Benign — Noncancerous.

Beta blockers — A drug option for men who need prostate surgery but have heart disease or are at risk of heart disease.

Biofeedback — Learning to control various automatic body functions such as heart rate, blood pressure, and temperature. Leads are placed on the body that are connected to a device which emits visual and sound clues when the desired change occurs. By observing these signals, the person can learn to produce the desired change voluntarily. Prostatodynia and incontinence can be treated with this technique.

Biopsy — Inserting a small needle through the rectum and up into the prostate to remove tissue samples. A pathologist will examine this tissue and look for cancer cells.

Bladder training — A technique for controlling incontinence. It teaches you to control your urges and gradually go longer and longer before urinating.

Bladder — A muscular pouch that temporarily stores urine until it can be excreted from your body.

Brachytherapy — A type of radiation used to treat prostate cancer in which 80 to 120 radioactive seeds are inserted into the prostate. The seeds are left in place permanently and continue to emit low levels of radiation for several months.

C

Castration — Surgical removal of the testicles.

Castrate range — The level of testosterone seen in men who've had their testicles removed.

Catheter — A slender, hollow tube used especially for draining urine from the bladder.

Central zone — The second-largest part of the prostate.

Chemotherapy — Special cell-killing drugs used to treat cancer.

Chronic bacterial prostatitis — A fairly rare condition that involves infection plus inflammation of the prostate. Although antibiotics can help, it usually takes much longer to clear up this infection than acute bacterial prostatitis. This condition also appears to be linked with repeated urinary tract infections (UTIs).

Chronic pelvic pain syndrome — The new term for nonbacterial prostatitis and prostatodynia.

Circumcision — Cutting off the foreskin of the penis.

Clinical stage — The stage your doctor believes your cancer to be in. He bases his estimation on the results of a variety of tests, which often include the DRE, PSA, TRUS, and a biopsy.

Clinical trial — Researchers use clinical trials to find out if promising new treatment methods really work. If you participate in one of these treatment studies, you will be given the new treatment and carefully watched. All your reactions will be written down and compared with others.

Collagen injections — Injecting collagen, the protein material found in connective tissue, into the area around the urethra to control incontinence.

Conformal radiation — A type of radiation that uses three-dimensional images and computers to direct delivery of radiation to treat prostate cancer. This allows the radiation beam to be targeted more precisely at the prostate and seminal vesicles, which means less damage to surrounding tissues.

Congestion (prostate congestion) — A buildup of prostatic fluid in the prostate. Can cause prostatosis.

Contact Visual Laser Ablation of the Prostate (CLAP) — A procedure involving direct contact of the laser fibers to the prostate tissue, using a tiny camera for guidance.

Cryosurgery — Also called cryosurgical ablation of the prostate (CSAP) or cryotherapy, this "ice cube" surgery attempts to eliminate cancer by freezing the cells to death.

D

DHEA — A hormone precursor that can be converted into testosterone in your body.

Digital rectal exam (DRE) — To check your prostate, your doctor will insert a gloved, lubricated finger into your rectum and press down. He will try to determine if your prostate has any hard lumps, which may suggest cancer, or if any areas feel tender and soft, which may indicate infection. A healthy prostate feels firm and elastic to the touch.

Dihydrotestosterone (DHT) — What testosterone is converted to once it reaches the prostate. This is the active form of testosterone in the prostate. The 5-alpha reductase enzymes are responsible for this conversion.

Durable power of attorney — A legal document that lets you appoint a trusted relative or friend to make business, property, asset, financial, and health decisions for you when you can't.

E

Ejaculation — The exit of semen from the body that normally occurs during sexual climax.

Ejaculatory duct — The channel formed by the ductus deferens and the seminal vesicle, which joins the prostatic urethra.

Epididymis — The storehouse for mature sperm. It also provides nutrition to immature sperm.

Epididymitis — Infection of the sperm ducts.

Erectile dysfunction — Consistently unable to become erect or stay erect long enough to have intercourse.

Estrogen — Female hormone that can stop testosterone from being produced by the testicles.

External beam radiation — A type of radiation therapy that bombards the general vicinity of the prostate in order to destroy the cancer cells.

External urethral sphincter — The muscle men use to control the release of urine.

F

Finasteride — One of the most prescribed medications for prostate problems. It works by slowing tissue growth and sometimes even shrinking your prostate to unblock your urethra. In addition, it blocks the conversion of testosterone to dihydrotestosterone, which tends to promote prostate enlargement. May help prevent prostate cancer. It is also used to treat cases of advanced prostate cancer.

Foley catheter — A special catheter inserted through the opening of the penis to drain urine from the bladder into a collection bag.

G

Gleason score — The most widely accepted cancer grading system. It is based on how cancer looks under the microscope. Cancers are classified as well-differentiated, moderately differentiated, or poorly differentiated. Poorly differentiated cancers are considered the most aggressive, which means the cancer is more likely to progress and spread throughout the body.

H

High intensity focused ultrasound (HIFU) — Uses highly controlled and concentrated ultrasound energy like a scalpel to treat BPH. This method focuses energy directly on the area that needs to be destroyed, sparing the surrounding healthy tissue. However, it usually causes temporary urinary retention and blood in the semen. Long-term effects are not known, and researchers suspect it may not be effective in men with large prostate glands.

Hormone therapy — Lowers male hormone levels to shrink or slow the progression of prostate cancer. Usually causes a loss of sexual desire and impotence.

I

Impotence — The inability to experience sexual intercourse, especially because of an inability to have an erection.

Incontinence — Inability to control the flow of urine.

Intermittent androgen suppression — A treatment option for advanced cancer that uses an LHRH agonist alone or with an antiandrogen to delay the prostate's take-over by deadly hormone-independent cells.

Interstitial Laser Coagulation of the Prostate (ILCP) — Ultrasound used to direct placement of laser fibers.

Interstitial radiation — See Brachytherapy.

K

Kegel exercises — Exercises to strengthen and tone the muscles that control urination. Many doctors recommend you begin these immediately after a radical prostatectomy. These exercises can also help treat impotence.

Kidneys — Where urine formation begins. Your body breaks down the food you eat into chemical byproducts which are transported by your bloodstream to the kidneys. The kidneys then filter your blood to collect the waste and excess water, forming urine.

L

Living will — A legal document used to spell out the type of medical treatment you want to receive if you have a terminal illness or become comatose. Also called a health care advance directive, or a directive to physicians. The medical staff must follow your directions exactly. Neither family wishes nor doctor beliefs can override your directives in states that recognize them. Laws concerning living wills vary from state to state.

Luteinizing hormone (LH) — A hormone produced by the pituitary gland. LH is responsible for telling the Leydig cells in your testicles to release testosterone into your bloodstream.

Luteinizing hormone-releasing hormone (LHRH) agonists — Drugs that prevent the release of or interfere with the action of male hormones. The most commonly used hormone therapy for prostate cancer, LHRH agonists shut off the supply of testosterone from the testicles by blocking the pituitary's production of LH. Sometimes referred to as medical orchiectomy.

Lycopene — A carotenoid associated with a reduced risk of prostate cancer. The substance in tomatoes that gives them their red color. Also found in watermelon, pink grapefruit, guava, papaya, apricots, and rose hips.

M

Mixed incontinence — A combination of incontinence symptoms. For men with an enlarged prostate, the most common combination is urge incontinence and overflow incontinence.

N

Neoadjuvant hormone therapy — Drugs to shut down the production of testosterone and prevent potential cancer spread. Generally, neoadjuvant hormone therapy is reserved for men with cancer that has spread into tissue right outside the prostate.

Nerve-sparing prostatectomy — Surgical technique that cuts close to the prostate, taking care to spare nearby nerves. This technique reduces the risk of impotence.

Nonbacterial prostatitis (NBP) — The most common type of prostatitis with inflammation in the prostate but no infection and no sign of bacteria. May or may not respond to antibiotics.

O

Oncologist — Doctor specially trained to diagnose and treat cancer.

Open prostatectomy — A type of surgery usually reserved for men who have very large prostates that make performing TURP or TUIP unsafe. It involves making an incision in the lower part of the stomach area and removing the prostate through the bladder or cutting directly into the prostate itself.

Orchiectomy — Surgical removal of the testicles.

Overflow incontinence — Occurs when an enlarged prostate presses against the urethra, blocking the flow of urine out of your body. Your bladder becomes too full, and small amounts of urine dribble out uncontrollably.

P

Paraurethral glands — Female glands near the urethra that are similar to the man's prostate. Just like the prostate, these glands can become inflamed and infected and even develop cancer.

Partin tables — Named after the Johns Hopkins doctor who created them, these tables combine information from your PSA level, your Gleason score, and your estimated clinical stage (based on the TNM system) to determine the pathological stage of your cancer. They tell you the likelihood that the cancer is still confined to your prostate or has spread beyond. Helpful for choosing a treatment strategy.

Pathological stage — The stage of your cancer, based on a pathologist's examination of actual prostate tissue or based on data from the Partin tables.

Pathologist — A doctor who specializes in diagnosing abnormal changes in tissue samples.

Patient-controlled analgesia (PCA) — An arrangement that allows you to control when you get pain medicine. When you begin to feel pain, you press a button to inject the medicine through an intravenous (IV) tube in your arm.

Pelvic pain syndrome — A combination of what were previously the separate categories of nonbacterial prostatitis and prostatodynia.

Penile clamp — A device used to control incontinence by squeezing the shaft of the penis so that no urine can flow through.

Penile cuff — A comfortable inflatable band that does much the same thing as the penile clamp.

Penile implants — In cases of impotence, a semirigid device can be surgically inserted into your penis to produce either a permanent erection or an erection that can be controlled by using a pump. Several different types of implants are available, ranging from a simple malleable rod to sophisticated hydraulic pump systems.

Penile self-injection — A shot of medicine designed to improve your ability to have an erection by increasing the flow of blood into your penis. Successfully reverses impotence except in those with extremely damaged blood vessels.

Penis — The organ of sexual intercourse. It is also the last and final passageway sperm or urine must pass through to exit the body.

Perineal radical prostatectomy — In this approach, the surgeon goes through the perineal region to reach the prostate. This is generally considered to be a less strenuous surgery so it may be used in older men or in men with poorer health who may have higher risks of complications. Used only for prostate cancer.

Perineum — The area between the penis and the anus.

Peripheral zone — The area making up the majority of the prostate.

Physician Data Query (PDQ) — A computer database of information from the National Cancer Institute.

Ploidy system — A system to grade cancer. This grading scale uses the number of complete chromosome sets in a cell to determine how dangerous or aggressive a cancer may be.

Pressure flow studies — This test measures the pressure in your bladder as you urinate. That number is then compared to the speed of your urine stream. Some doctors feel this test is the best way to find out how much your ability to urinate is affected. A small tube called a catheter is inserted into your penis, through the urethra, and into your bladder. This study will confirm whether or not you will benefit from surgery.

Priaprism — Prolonged erection that can cause permanent damage to your penis.

Prostascint — This test can accurately detect cancer spread outside the prostate. A harmless radioactive particle is injected, which then reveals the exact location of all prostate cancer in the body during a whole-body scan.

Prostatalgia — Another term for prostatodynia.

Prostate gland — The part-muscle, part-gland structure that produces nutrient-rich secretions that combine with sperm to make semen.

Prostate massage — Rubbing the prostate to help drain it and increase blood flow to it.

Prostate specific antigen (PSA) — PSA is a protein that is secreted into your prostatic ducts during ejaculation. The main purpose of PSA is to liquefy semen after ejaculation so sperm may be released on their journey to find an available egg to fertilize. Since the early 1990s, doctors have used PSA to test for prostate cancer.

Prostate specific antigen (PSA) test — Measures your levels of PSA. High PSA levels signal you have a problem with your prostate. Your doctor may use this test to confirm his suspicions of either BPH or prostate cancer.

Prostate stones — Similar to stones found in the gallbladder or kidneys, these are one of the main causes of a prostate infection that fails to respond to treatment. Prostate stones are normally harmless unless they harbor bacteria. Then, they serve as a breeding ground for repeated infections.

Prostatectomy — Prostate surgery. A prostatectomy for BPH removes all the tissue inside the prostate, leaving only the prostatic capsule. A prostatectomy for prostate cancer removes the entire prostate.

Prostatic capsule — The muscular tissue enclosing the entire prostate.

Prostatic fluid — The thin liquid secreted by the prostate that combines with sperm to make semen.

Prostatic intraepithelial neoplasia (PIN) — Abnormal cells that have a strong link to cancer. If your biopsy points out PIN, you should have another one. About half the time another biopsy will find cancer.

Prostatic urethra — The part of the urethra completely encircled by the prostate gland.

Prostatic — Having to do with the prostate gland.

Prostatism — Any prostate problem that interferes with urine flow from the bladder. Traditionally, all lower urinary tract symptoms in older men were called prostatism.

Prostatitis — An inflamed prostate gland, which may or may not be infected. Prostatitis is a general term that includes infections, inflammation, and nonbacterial conditions of the prostate. There are three types of prostatitis: acute bacterial prostatitis, chronic bacterial prostatitis, and chronic nonbacterial prostatitis.

Prostatodynia — A painful prostate with no apparent signs of inflammation or infection. A few cases respond well to antibiotics. Researchers speculate prostatodynia may be caused by spasms of the bladder, pelvic, or rectal muscles.

Prostatomegaly — Enlargement of the prostate gland.

Prostatosis — Any problem with the prostate that isn't cancer or an inflammatory condition. This term is often used interchangeably with the term noninfectious prostatitis. Some doctors prefer prostatosis over nonbacterial prostatitis because of the possibility that bacteria may one day be linked to nonbacterial prostatitis.

PSA density (PSAD) — This measurement is useful for distinguishing men with BPH from men with prostate cancer. It is determined by dividing your PSA number by the volume of your prostate. The higher your PSA density, the greater your risk of cancer.

PSA velocity (PSAV) — Also known as serial PSA testing, the velocity measures annual changes in PSA levels.

Pulmonary embolism — A blood clot that plugs the arteries supplying blood to the lungs. One of the possible complications of prostate surgery, especially an open prostatectomy.

R

Radiation therapy (radiotherapy) — The use of high-energy waves to stop the progress of prostate cancer by interfering with cancer cell reproduction. Radiation is a good option when the cancer has penetrated the prostate capsule but has only spread to surrounding tissue.

Radical prostatectomy — Surgical procedure that removes the entire prostate gland.

Residual urine test — This procedure is designed to show if the bladder empties normally or not. A catheter is inserted into the bladder to empty and measure any remaining urine.

Retrograde ejaculation — When semen backs up into the bladder instead of being forced out through the penis. This renders most men infertile but should not interfere with the sensation of orgasm. Also called "dry ejaculation."

Retropubic prostatectomy — The most common type of radical prostatectomy. The surgeon cuts into the lower section of your abdominal area behind the pubic bone to get to your prostate. This approach may be used for either open prostatectomy (for BPH) or radical prostatectomy (for prostate cancer).

S

Scrotum — The sac of skin that contains the testicles.

Semen — The fluid containing sperm which comes out of the penis during sexual excitement.

Seminal vesicles — Small sacs connected to the ductus deferens that produce nutrient-rich secretions that combine with sperm to make semen.

Sperm — A reproductive cell capable of fertilizing a woman's egg, which, if timing is right and conditions are good, may eventually develop into a baby.

Sphincter — A ring-shaped muscle that surrounds various openings in the body and can control its opening and closing by contracting or expanding.

Spinal cord compression — If your cancer has spread to the lower vertebrae of the spine, you may experience pressure on your spine causing extreme weakness in your lower body and difficulty in controlling bowel movements. This is a serious problem which can lead to paralysis. Treatment may include hormone therapy, bilateral orchiectomy, steroids, or surgery.

Staging — A way of categorizing the different levels of cancer development.

Stents — To ease obstructed urinary flow, a plastic or metal device is inserted through the urethra to the narrowed area and allowed to expand like a spring. Stents can be inserted quickly, require little recovery time, do not affect sexual functioning, and may eliminate the need for a catheter.

Stress incontinence — Urine leakage triggered by coughing, sneezing, or straining. This usually happens when the muscle that controls urine flow, the bladder sphincter, becomes weak.

Suprapubic prostatectomy — A prostatectomy where the surgeon goes through your bladder to reach your prostate. This approach is only used for BPH.

T

Testicles — The two oval glands suspended in the scrotum that make sperm and testosterone.

Testosterone — A male steroid sex hormone, produced in the testicles and adrenal glands. Affects the growth of prostate tissue.

Timed voiding — A set schedule for urination that keeps your bladder emptied regularly and cuts the risk of involuntary leakage.

Total incontinence — A complete inability to control urine.

Transcutaneous electrical nerve stimulation (TENS) — A pain relief option using mild electrical stimulation on your skin. This system provides nondrug relief by interfering with pain's pathway to your brain.

Transition zone — The smallest area of the prostate, making up only 5 to 10 percent of the entire gland.

Transrectal ultrasonography (TRUS) — During this procedure, a probe is inserted about 3 to 4 inches into your rectum. The probe makes images of your prostate and surrounding tissues as it is being removed. Your urologist will use TRUS to determine the size of your prostate and identify areas that may be cancerous. If your doctor decides a biopsy is needed, he will use TRUS to help him guide the biopsy needle.

Transurethral incision of the prostate (TUIP) — An endoscopic surgical procedure limited to men with smaller prostates in which an instrument is passed through the urethra to make one or two cuts in the prostate and prostate capsule, reducing constriction of the urethra. This procedure can be done on an outpatient basis.

Transurethral microwave thermotherapy (TUMT) — An experimental procedure that involves sending computer-regulated microwave heat through a catheter to selected portions of the prostate to destroy excess prostate tissue. Because of the device's design, it can only be used in men with medium-sized prostates. Also, it may take six weeks to three months for changes to become significantly noticeable.

Transurethral needle ablation (TUNA) — A type of heat therapy that uses radio frequency energy to destroy excess prostate tissue. TUNA seems to work best in men who have slight obstructions.

Transurethral resection of the prostate (TUR or TURP) — Surgical removal of the prostate's inner portion by an endoscopic approach through the urethra, with no external incision. This is the most common treatment for symptomatic BPH and usually requires a hospital stay.

Transurethral suppository — Alprostadil, an impotence drug, is delivered into the tip of your penis with a syringe-type applicator.

Transurethral vaporization of the prostate (TVP) — This procedure is similar to TURP, but instead of cutting away excess tissue, an electric current vaporizes the extra tissue. TVP involves a shorter hospital stay and perhaps less risk of bleeding, incontinence, or narrowing of the urethra.

Tumor, Node, Metastases (TNM) system — A system for staging cancer. T indicates the size and spread of cancer within and near the prostate; N indicates if and where the cancer has spread to the lymph nodes; M indicates that cancer has spread to other organs and sites in the body.

U

Ureters — Two tubes, attached to the center of each kidney, that transport urine to the bladder.

Urethra — The tube that carries urine from the bladder through the penis and out of the body. It also carries semen from the prostatic urethra out of the body.

Urethral stricture — A problem that occurs when scar tissue from an injury or untreated infection in the urethra shrinks, causing the urethra to narrow and sometimes become shorter. This makes it difficult and painful to urinate or ejaculate. Surgery is often necessary to correct this problem.

Urethritis — An inflammation of the urethra. It may be caused by an infection, an irritation, or a minor injury.

Urethrocystoscopy — Using a special tool inserted through the penis tip and up into the urethra, this test allows your doctor to examine your urethra and bladder before he actually performs surgery in your prostate. What he sees helps him determine the best treatment approach.

Urge incontinence — Difficulty controlling urination possibly caused by a prostate infection or a prostatectomy. You feel the sudden need to urinate, but can't reach the bathroom in time.

Urinary (urethral) sphincter — The muscle that controls urine flow.

Urinary retention — Incomplete emptying of the bladder.

Uroflowmetry — Another name for the uroflow test. Simple and painless, all you need is a full bladder. You urinate into a special toilet, which measures how much urine you pass and records the speed of your urine stream.

Urologist — A doctor who specializes in treating disorders of the urinary system and male reproductive system.

V

Vacuum pump — This nonsurgical option for treating impotence uses a vacuum to pull blood into the penis. Once fully erect, a rubber ring is placed at the base of the penis to retain the blood until intercourse is completed.

Vas deferens — The system of tubes that conveys the sperm from the testicles to the penis.

Vasectomy — A form of male birth control which either ties or removes the vas deferens so that sperm cannot pass through.

Visual laser ablation of the prostate (VLAP) — One of the new laser prostatectomy techniques currently being tested. The equipment combines a laser and a tiny camera which projects a picture onto a television monitor. This lets the doctor direct the laser beam precisely into the prostate. The high temperatures kill the extra prostate tissue, which is gradually shed by the prostate over the next couple of weeks and is either absorbed by the body or washed away in the urine.

Visualization — A technique to help control body processes by using a picture in your mind. You can learn different ways to soothe, heal, calm, or control your body.

Volume monitors — Specialized nerves in the trigone (base of bladder) and bladder wall that monitor the amount of urine in the bladder. Once enough liquid has collected, they signal the brain that the bladder needs to be emptied.

W

Watchful waiting — Merely monitoring prostate symptoms carefully while postponing treatment for as long as possible.

Whitmore-Jewett system — A system for staging cancer, also known as the ABCD staging system. Stages may range from stage A, where the tumor is still tiny and confined to the prostate, to stage D, where cancer has spread to the lymph nodes or to other organs outside the prostate. The lower the stage, the more likely the cancer can be cured. Stage D tumors are not usually curable.

Bibliography

Introduction
CA — A Cancer Journal for Clinicians (47,4:239)
Cancer (77,7:1342)
Prostate Cancer Information, American Cancer Society, Internet WWW
  address <http://www.cancer.org/statistics/97cff/97prosta.html>
  retrieved on February 13, 1998

Chapter 1
Epidemiology of Prostate Disease, Springer-Verlag, Berlin, Germany, 1995
Herbal Prescriptions for Better Health, Prima Publishing, Rocklin, Calif.,
  1996
Overcoming Bladder Disorders, HarperCollins Publishers, New York, 1990
Prostate Health Watch, Michigan State University, Internet WWW address
  <http://www.msu.edu/user/prostate/phw/whatis.html> retrieved on
  Feb. 13, 1998
Sexual Trivia, Internet WWW address <http://www.village.com.au/
  airwaves/austereo/pillow/trivia.htm> retrieved on Feb.13, 1998
The American Medical Association Encyclopedia of Medicine, Random
  House, New York, 1989
The Anatomy Coloring Book, HarperCollins Publishers, New York, 1993
*The Columbia University College of Physicians and Surgeons Complete
  Home Medical Guide*, Crown Publishers, Inc., New York, 1995
The Compass in Your Nose and Other Astonishing Facts About Humans,
  Jeremy P. Tarcher, Inc., Los Angeles, 1989
The Reader's Digest Book of Facts, Pleasantville, N.Y., 1995

Chapter 2
American Health (15,4:70)
Doctor Shopping, Health Information Press, Los Angeles, Calif., 1996
Examining Your Doctor, Carol Publishing Group, New York, 1995
Get the Facts on Anyone, Macmillan, New York, 1995
Medical Care (33,12:1176)
"Medicare Coverage for Second Surgical Opinions," Publication No. HCFA
  02173, U.S. Department of Health and Human Services, Health Care
  Financing Administration, 200 Independence Ave., S.W., Room 428H,
  Washington, D.C. 20201
Postgraduate Medicine (100,6:31)
Prostate Cancer: A Survivor's Guide, Seneca House Press, New Port
  Richey, Fla., 1996
*The Columbia University College of Physicians and Surgeons Complete
  Home Medical Guide*, Crown Publishers, Inc., New York, 1995
The Informer (Spring/Summer 1993)
The New England Journal of Medicine (324,6:370 and 377)
The Wall Street Journal (July 9, 1993, B1)
*Top Secret Information the Government, Banks, and Retailers Don't Want
  You to Know*, FC&A Publishing, Peachtree City, Ga., 1996
"What Will Your Operation Cost?" American College of Surgeons, 55 East
  Erie Street, Chicago, IL 60611

"Who Should Do Your Operation?" American College of Surgeons, 55 East Erie Street, Chicago, IL 60611

"1997 Guide to Health Insurance for People with Medicare," Publication No. HCFA 02110, Health Care Financing Administration, 7500 Security Boulevard, Baltimore, Md. 21244-1850

Chapter 3

American Family Physician (54,5:1704)

Archivio Italiano di Urologica, Nefrologia, Andrologia (63,3:341)

British Journal of Urology (64,5:496 and 71,4:433)

Cecil Textbook of Diseases, Harcourt Brace Jovanovich, Philadelphia, 1992

Complementary Therapies in Medicine (4,1:21)

Current Opinion in Urology (6,1:53)

Epidemiology of Prostate Disease, Springer-Verlag, Berlin, 1995

European Urology (29,1:111)

Hinyokika Kiyo (34,3:561)

Journal of Autoimmunity (10,2:107)

Journal of Clinical Microbiology (34,12:3120)

Journal of Steroid Biochemistry and Molecular Biology (43,6:557)

Natural Health, Natural Medicine: A Comprehensive Manual for Wellness and Self-care, Houghton Mifflin Co., New York, 1995

Postgraduate Medicine (100,6:31)

Prostate Problems, Dr. Walt Stoll, Internet WWW address<http://www.bcn.net/~stoll/prostate.html> retrieved on February 13, 1998

Prostatic Outflow Obstruction: Clinical Investigation and Treatment, Blackwell Science, Oxford, England, 1994

Prostatitis: Disorders of the Prostate, The National Institute of Diabetes and Digestive and Kidney Diseases, Internet WWW address <http://www.niddk.nih.gov/kusums/prstitis.htm> retrieved on February 13, 1998

Prostatitis Frequently Asked Questions, Ron Kinner, Internet WWW address <http://prostate.org/prosfaq.html> retrieved on June 30, 1997

Spontaneous Healing, Random House, New York, 1995

The American Medical Association Encyclopedia of Medicine, Random House, New York, 1989

Complete Guide to Symptoms, Illness & Surgery, The Berkley Publishing Group, New York, 1995

The American Medical Association Family Medical Guide, Random House, New York, 1994

The Journal of the American Medical Association (274,11:868)

The Journal of Urology (154,4:1378; 155,4:1301; 155,3:961; 155,6:1950; and 157,3:863)

The Lancet (347,9017:1711)

The Prostate Book, W.W. Norton & Co., New York, 1994

The Western Journal of Medicine (164,5:435)

U.S. Pharmacist (22,6:47)

Chapter 4

American Journal of Epidemiology (142,9:965)

Are You Normal?, St. Martin's Press, New York, 1995

Better Nutrition (58,8:54)

British Journal of Urology (78,3:325 and 81,3:383)

British Medical Journal (313,7072:1569)

Cancer Fighting Foods, Jeffrey S. Bland, Ph.D., Internet WWW address <http://www.newhope.com:80/magazines/delicious/D_backs/Sep_97/nat_heal.html> retrieved on February 17, 1998

HerbalGram (34:12 and 40:18)

Herbal Prescriptions for Better Health, Prima Publishing, Rocklin, Calif., 1996

Herbs for Health (Spring/Summer 1996)

Herbs of Choice: The Therapeutic Use of Phytomedicinals, Varro E. Tyler, Ph.D., Sc.D., The Hayworth Press, Binghamton, N.Y., 1994

Infections in Urology (10,4:118)

Journal of Endocrinology (147:295-302)

Journal of the Maine Medical Association (49,3:99)

McConnell JD, Barry MJ, Bruskewitz RC, et al. *Benign Prostatic Hyperplasia: Diagnosis and Treatment*. Clinical Practice Guideline, Number 8. AHCPR Publication No. 94-0582. Rockville, MD: Agency for Health Care Policy and Research, Public Health Service, U.S. Department of Health and Human Services. February 1994

Medical Tribune for the Family Physician (35,4:1 and 36,1:16)

Medical Update (20,1:5)

Patient Outcomes Research Team — Prostate Disease, Project Period: September 1, 1989 - August 31, 1994, Final Report, National Technical Information Service, Springfield, Va. 22161

Pharmacy Times (61,2:41)

Prostate Enlargement: Benign Prostatic Hyperplasia, National Institute of Diabetes and Digestive and Kidney Disorders of the National Institutes of Health, Internet WWW address <http://www.niddk.nih.gov/ProstateEnlargement/ProstateEnlargement.html> retrieved on February 17, 1998

Prostate Patients Should Take More Active Role in Treatment Strategy, Doctor's Guide to Medical and Other News, Internet WWW address <http://www.pslgroup.com/dg/5cfe.htm> retrieved on February 17, 1998

The Atlanta Journal/Constitution (Dec. 23, 1997, A1)

The Columbia University College of Physicians and Surgeons Complete Home Medical Guide, Crown Publishers, Inc., New York, 1995

The Doctor's Complete Guide to Vitamins and Minerals, Dell Publishing Group, Inc., New York, 1994

The Honest Herbal, by Varro E. Tyler, Ph.D., Haworth Press, Inc., Binghamton, N.Y., 1993

The Journal of Urology (154:174-180)

The New England Journal of Medicine (332,2:99 and 107; 335,8:533; 335,11:823; 338,9:557 and 612)

Treating Your Enlarged Prostate, U.S. Department of Health and Human Services, Public Health Service, Agency for Health Care Policy and Research, Executive Office Center, Suite 501, 2101 East Jefferson St., Rockville, Md. 20852

Urologic Clinics of North America (22,2:407)

Urology (48,1:12 and 49:839)

U.S. Pharmacist (22,6:17)

Visualization for Change, 2nd ed., New Harbinger Publications, Inc., Oakland, Ca., 1994

Drugs and Aging (9,5:379)

Chapter 5
AORN Journal (61,5:807)
British Journal of Urology (77,3:391 and 79,2:172,177)
Canadian Medical Association Journal (150,9:1449)
Emergency Medicine (28,5:86)
Examining Your Doctor, Carol Publishing Group, New York, 1995
Food and Drug Administration news release (P96-9), May 6, 1996
Health After 50 (9,9:8)
McConnell JD, Barry MJ, Bruskewitz RC, et al. *Benign Prostatic Hyperplasia: Diagnosis and Treatment.* Clinical Practice Guideline, Number 8. AHCPR Publication No. 94-0582. Rockville, MD: Agency for Health Care Policy and Research, Public Health Service, U.S. Department of Health and Human Services. February 1994.
Minutes, Medicare and Medicaid Agency, Internet WWW address <http://www.hcfa.gov> retrieved on Dec. 19, 1997
Journal of Endourology (11,3:197)
Journal of Urology (156,2, Part 1:413)
Natural Medicines and Cures Your Doctor Never Tells You About, FC&A Publishing, Peachtree City, Ga., 1995
Neurourology and Urodynamics (15,6:619)
Pain Control After Surgery. A Patient's Guide, AHCPR Publication No. 92-0021, U.S. Department of Health and Human Services, Public Health Service, Agency for Health Care Policy and Research, Executive Office Center, Suite 501, 2101 East Jefferson St., Rockville, Md. 20852
Postgraduate Medicine (94,6:141)
Prostate Enlargement: Benign Prostatic Hyperplasia, National Institute of Diabetes and Digestive and Kidney Disorders of the National Institutes of Health, Internet WWW address <http://www.niddk.nih.gov/ProstateEnlargement/ProstateEnlargement.html> retrieved on April 1, 1997
Textbook of Benign Prostatic Hyperplasia, Isis Medical Media, Oxford, UK, 1996
The Big Book of Health Tips, FC&A Publishing, Peachtree City, Ga., 1996
The Journal of the American Medical Association (266,4:459)
The New England Journal of Medicine (332,2:99)
The Surgery Book: An Illustrated Guide to 73 of the Most Common Operations, St. Martin's Press, New York, 1993
Transfusion (34,2:110)
Treating Your Enlarged Prostate, AHCPR Publication No. 94-0584, U.S. Department of Health and Human Services, Public Health Service, Agency for Health Care Policy and Research, Executive Office Center, Suite 501, 2101 East Jefferson St., Rockville, Md. 20852
Ultrasound in Medicine and Biology (22,2:193)
Urologic Clinics of North America (23,4:623)

Chapter 6
Anesthesia for Ambulatory Surgery, American Society of Anesthesiologists, 520 N. Northwest Highway, Park Ridge, Ill. 60068-2573
Archives of Internal Medicine (157:1026-1030)
Be Careful What You Pray For ... You Just Might Get It, HarperCollins Publishers, New York, 1997

Be Informed: Learning more about your operation will help you make better decisions about your health care, AHCPR Pub. No. 95-0027, Agency for Health Care Policy and Research, Executive Office Center, Suite 501, 2101 East Jefferson Street, Rockville, Md. 20852

British Journal of Urology (80,1:111)

Canadian Medical Association Journal (150,9:1449)

Examining Your Doctor, Carol Publishing Group, New York, 1995

Know Your Anesthesiologist, American Society of Anesthesiologists, 520 N. Northwest Highway, Park Ridge, Ill. 60068-2573

Natural Healing Newsletter (7,81:8)

Natural Medicines and Cures Your Doctor Never Tells You About, FC&A Publishing, Peachtree City, Ga., 1995

Pain Control After Surgery. A Patient's Guide, AHCPR Pub. No. 92-0021, Agency for Health Care Policy and Research, Executive Office Center, Suite 501, 2101 East Jefferson St., Rockville, Md. 20852

The Big Book of Health Tips, FC&A Publishing, Peachtree City, Ga., 1996

Transfusion (34,2:110)

The Mozart Effect, Avon Books, New York, 1997

The New England Journal of Medicine (332,2:99 and 335,23:1713)

Chapter 7

American Journal of Epidemiology (143,7:692)

British Journal of Urology (77:481-493)

Cancer (64,3:598)

Cancer Epidemiology, Biomarkers & Prevention (5,7:509)

"Diet, Nutrition, and Prostate Cancer," American Institute for Cancer Research, 1759 R Street, N.W., Washington, D.C. 20069

Environmental Health Perspectives (104,5:478)

Geriatrics (51,5:61)

Interview with Professor Peter Bramley, Division of Biochemistry, Royal Holloway Hospital, University of London, Egham, England, November 14, 1997

Journal of the American College of Nutrition (16,2:109)

Journal of the American Medical Association (278,18:1509)

Journal of the National Cancer Institute (87,9:662 and 89,24:1881)

Medical Tribune for the Internist and Cardiologist (35,24:1)

Medicine and Science in Sports and Exercise (28,1:97)

Prostate (4,4:345)

"Prostate Cancer Prevention Trial Recruitment of 18,000 Men Completed," National Cancer Institute, Internet WWW address <http://www.graylab.ac.uk/cancernet/600047.html> retrieved on February 18, 1998

Prostate Cancer: Risk Associated with Environmental Substances, Dr. K.J. Aronson, et.al, 1998

Science (274:1371-1374 and 279,5350:563)

Science News (145,8:145; 149,4:61; and 151,8:126)

The Journal of Urology (154:404)

Chapter 8

American Family Physician (56,5:1450)

Annals of Internal Medicine (125,2:118)

Archives of Family Medicine (6,1:72)

British Journal of Urology (77:851)
Canadian Medical Association Journal (153,7:935)
FDA Consumer (28,10:5)
Geriatrics (49,7:52)
Important Information About Prostate-Specific Antigen (PSA), The Prostate
    Health Council, 300 West Pratt Street, Suite 401, Baltimore, Md. 21201
Journal of Urology (143,3:587)
Mayo Clinic Proceedings (72:337)
New Prostate Test on the Horizon, Reuters, Internet WWW address
    <http://www.shn.net/cgi-bin/gen.cgi?page=Article&id=Reuters_
    t0205-1f.txt&source=Reuters> retrieved on March 2, 1998
Postgraduate Medicine (100,3:90 and 100,6:31)
Prostate Cancer Screening, Wesley Eastridge, M.D., Internet WWW
    address <http://kpt1.tricon.net/Personal/wesley/prostate> retrieved
    on Feb. 4, 1998
*Q&A About the Prostate, Lung, Colorectal, and Ovarian Cancer Screening
    Trial*, Sapient Health Network, Internet WWW address
    <http://www.shn. net/cgi-bin/gen.cgi?page=Article&id=nws_
    Q_n_A_About_980227_3183. html> retrieved on March 2, 1998
Science News (139,17:261 and 151,16:240)
Scientific American (September 1996)
The Journal of the American Medical Association (267,16:2227,2236;
    276,23:1904; and 277,18:1452,1456,1475)
The Journal of Urology (147,3:810 and 155,2:607)
The Lancet (347,9010:1250)
The New England Journal of Medicine (335,5:304,345 and 337,25:1849)
Urology (47,4:511)

Chapter 9
50 Essential Things to Do When the Doctor Says It's Cancer, Penguin
    Books, New York, 1993
Annals of Internal Medicine (125,2:118))
British Medical Journal (6931,308:780)
Cancer (73,11:2791 and 79,10:1977)
Diet, Nutrition, and Prostate Cancer, American Institute for Cancer
    Research, 1759 R Street, N.W., Washington, D.C. 20069
Doubt Cast on Nerve-Sparing Prostate Surgery, Denise Mann, Internet
    WWW address <http://nytsyn.com:80/live/Week/220_080897_
    120012_16977.html> retrieved on Aug. 11, 1997
Emergency Medicine (28,5:86)
Epidemiology of Prostate Disease, Springer-Verlag, Berlin, Germany, 1995
FDA Consumer (28,10:5)
Infections in Urology (10,3:70)
Journal of Clinical Oncology (1997,15:1478)
Journal of the Canadian Medical Association (153,7:935)
Journal of the National Cancer Institute (88,3/4:166)
Looking for Prostate Cancer, Internet WWW address
    <http://www.shn.net/cgi-bin/gen.cgi?page=Article&id=nws_Looking
    _for_980123_2971.html&source=Article> retrieved on March 2, 1998
Modern Medicine (65,11)
National Cancer Institute, Office of Cancer Communications, 31 Center

Drive, MSC 2580, Bethesda, Md. 20892-2580

Patient Outcomes Research Team — Prostate Disease, Project Period: September 1, 1989 - August 31, 1994, Final Report, National Technical Information Service, Springfield, Va. 22161

Postgraduate Medicine (100,3:105 and 100,3:125)

Postprostatectomy Radiation Does Not Cause Urinary Incontinence, Internet WWW address <http://www.shn.net/cgi-bin/gen.cgi?page= Article&id=Reuters_c101158f.nws&source=Reuters> retrieved on Jan. 23, 1998

Prostate Cancer Information, American Cancer Society, Internet WWW address <http://www.cancer.org/prostate/prask.html> retrieved on July 7, 1997

Prostate Cancer Resource Guide, American Foundation for Urologic Disease, Inc., 300 West Pratt Street, Suite 401, Baltimore, Md. 21201

Prostate Cancer Surgery Beneficial, Internet WWW address <http://www.pathfinder.com/@@1934iQYA3t1OEyjz/living/latest/RB> retrieved on July 3, 1997

Prostate Cancer Treatment, Prostate Health Watch (1,1:5)

Prostate Cancer: What Every Man Over 40 Should Know, The Prostate Health Council, 300 West Pratt Street, Suite 401, Baltimore, MD 21201

Radiation After Prostatectomy Beneficial for Patients With Elevated PSA, Internet WWW address <http://www.shn.net/cgi-bin/gen.cgi?page= Article&id=Reuters_cl09257b.nws&source=Reuters> retrieved on Nov. 16, 1997

Radical Surgery Not Cure Cancer, Internet WWW address <http://www. wdn.com/mirkin/6690.html> retrieved on Sept. 22, 1997

Report on The Management of Clinically Localized Prostate Cancer, The American Urological Association, 1120 North Charles St., Baltimore, Md. 21201-1566

Seed Therapy Shows Success in Improving Quality of Life for Prostate Cancer Patients at UCSF, Internet WWW address <http://www.business-wire.com:80/cgi-bin/sr_headline.sh?/bw.091097/471931> retrieved on Sept. 11, 1997

Side effects can hit hard, Richard Saltus, Internet WWW address <http://www.boston.com:80/dailyglobe/globehtml/012/Side_effects_ca n_hit_hard.htm> retrieved on Jan. 12, 1998

The Boston Globe (Jan. 12, 1998, C2)

The Journal of the American Medical Association (273,2:129; 274,1:69; 277,18:1445; 278,1:44; and 278,21:1727)

The Journal of Urology (150,1:110; 154:2144; and 156, 5:1696)

The Lancet (349,9056:906 and 349,9066:1681)

The New England Journal of Medicine (337,5:295)

The Prostate Book, W.W. Norton & Co., New York, 1994

Urology for the House Officer, Williams and Wilkins, Baltimore, Md., 1995

When Your Doctor Doesn't Know Best, Simon & Schuster, New York, 1995

Chapter 10

50 Essential Things to Do When the Doctor Says It's Cancer, Penguin Books, New York, 1993

801 Prescription Drugs: Good Effects, Side Effects & Natural Healing Alternatives, FC&A Publishing, Peachtree City, Ga., 1996

American Journal of Clinical Nutrition (66,2:398 and 66,2:425)

HerbalGram (40:17)

Herbs for Health (2,5:71)

Men Needed for Prostate Cancer Study, Internet WWW address <http://www.newhope.com:80/public/delicious/D%21_backs/Jun_97/prostate.html> retrieved on June 12, 1997

New Evidence on Old Vitamin: Vitamin D May Combat Breast, Colon, and Prostate Cancer, Ralph W. Moss, Ph.D., Internet WWW address <http://www.ralphmoss.com/vitaminD.html> retrieved on January 13, 1998

Science News (147,9:134)

Soyfoods USA (1,2)

Study Drowns Anti-Cancer Hype of Shark Cartilage, Jacqueline Stenson, Internet WWW address <http://nytsyn.com:80/live/Week/139_051997_154215_25810.html> retrieved on May 22, 1997

Super LifeSpan, Super Health, FC&A Publishing, Peachtree City, Ga., 1997

Chapter 11

British Medical Journal (6931:308:780)

Cancer Research (57,13:2559)

Fabulous Fallacies, Crown Publishers, New York, 1982

Important Information About Prostate-Specific Antigen (PSA), The Prostate Health Council, 300 West Pratt Street, Suite 401, Baltimore, MD 21201

Medical Tribune (38,5:1997)

New Perspectives in Cancer Diagnosis and Management (2,1:1994)

Overcoming Bladder Disorders, HarperPerennial, New York, 1990

Postgraduate Medicine (100,3:139)

Proceedings of the National Academy of Sciences (94,15:8099)

Prostate Cancel Labeling Expanded for Novantrone, Internet WWW address <http://www.prnewswire.com:80/cgi-bin/stories.pl?ACCT=104&STORY=/oracle/dbtmp/> retrieved on June 13, 1997

Prostate Cancer Treatment, Prostate Health Watch (1,1)

Report on The Management of Clinically Localized Prostate Cancer, The American Urological Association Prostate Cancer Clinical Guidelines Panel, The American Urological Association, 1995

Shape Your Health Care Future with Health Care Advance Directives, Internet WWW address <http://www.ama-assn.org/public/booklets/livgwill.htm> retrieved on April 6, 1998

The Journal of the American Medical Association (274,1:69 and 277,20:1580)

The New England Journal of Medicine (337,5:295)

Top Secret Information the Government, Banks, and Retailers Don't Want You to Know, FC&A Publishing, Peachtree City, Ga., 1996

Urology and the Primary Care Practitioner, Mosby-Wolfe Medical Communications, London, England, 1995

Urology for the House Officer, Williams and Wilkins, Baltimore, Md., 1995

Chapter 12

American Family Physician (54,2:683 and 54,5:1661)

Annals of Internal Medicine (103,4:507)

Archives of Internal Medicine (156:545)

Consumer Reports (October 1997)
Geriatrics (51,4:47 and 51,6:18)
Hospital Pharmacy Times (62,5:5HPT)
Journal of Urology (155:1256)
Overcoming Bladder Disorders, HarperPerennial, N.Y., 1991
Postgraduate Medicine (97,5:109 and 100,3:129)
Symptoms, Bantam Books, New York, 1989

Chapter 13
American Family Physician (55,5:1902 and 55,5:1967)
Ancient Healing, Publications International Ltd., Lincolnwood, Ill., 1997
British Journal of Urology (71,1:52)
British Medical Journal (312,7035:859 and 312,7045:1512)
Herbs of Choice, The Hayworth Press, Binghamton, N.Y., 1994
Impotence: A guide for men with diabetes, Publication No. 81115A, Impotence
    Information Center, Department D, P.O. Box 9, Minneapolis, Minn.
    55440
Male Impotence: A Treatment Guide, The Geddings Osbon Foundation,
    P.O. Box 1593, Augusta, Ga. 30903
Medical Tribune (38,20:36)
Medical Update (20,1:5)
Modern Medicine (59,9:63)
Newsweek (130,20:62)
*Overcoming Impotence: A Doctor's Proven Guide to Regaining Sexual Vitali-
    ty*, Prentice-Hall, Englewood Cliffs, N.J., 1994
Postgraduate Medicine (100,3:133)
"Report on the Treatment of Organic Erectile Dysfunction," American
    Urological Association, Inc., 1120 North Charles St., Baltimore, Md.
    21201-5559
*The Columbia University College of Physicians and Surgeons Complete
    Home Medical Guide*, Crown Publishers, Inc., New York, 1995
The New England Journal of Medicine (336,1:1)

Chapter 14
Looking for Prostate Cancer Q&A, Salma Khan, MD, Internet WWW
    address <http://www.shn.net/cgi-bin/gen.cgi?page=Article&id=
    nws_Looking_for_980123_2971.html&source=Article> retrieved on
    March 2, 1998
McConnell JD, Barry MJ, Bruskewitz RC, et al. *Benign Prostatic Hyperpla-
    sia: Diagnosis and Treatment*, Clinical Practice Guideline, Number 8.
    AHCPR Publication No. 94-0582. Rockville, MD: Agency for Health Care
    Policy and Research, Public Health Service, U.S. Department of Health
    and Human Services. February 1994.
Treating Your Enlarged Prostate, U.S. Department of Health and Human
    Services, Public Health Service, Agency for Health Care Policy and
    Research, Executive Office Center, Suite 501, 2101 East Jefferson St.,
    Rockville, Md. 20852
Urology, Williams & Wilkins, Baltimore, Md., 1995

Chapter 15
American Cancer Society, Internet WWW address <http://www.cancer.

org/bottomcancinfo.html> retrieved on March 18, 1988
National Institute of Diabetes and Digestive and Kidney Diseases, Internet WWW address <http://www.niddk.nih.gov/> retrieved on March 18, 1998
"Who to Call," Prostate Cancer Resource Network, P.O. Box 966, New Port Richey, Fla. 34656

Chapter 16
801 Prescription Drugs: Good Effects, Side Effects & Natural Healing Alternatives, FC&A Publishing, Peachtree City, Ga., 1996
Current Opinion in Urology (6,1:53)
Epidemiology of Prostate Disease, Springer-Verlag, Berlin, 1995
"Novantrone Information," Immunex, Internet WWW address <http://www.immunex.com/PRODUCTS/HTML/novandefault.html> retrieved on March 18, 1998
Prostate Cancer Resource Guide, American Foundation for Urologic Disease, Inc., 300 West Pratt Street, Suite 401, Baltimore, Md. 21201
U.S. Pharmacist (22,6:47)
Urology (43,4:460)

Index